The Physician's Guide to Disease Management

Patient-Centered Care for the 21st Century

James B. Couch, MD, JD, FACPE
Director, Disease Management Consulting
Coopers & Lybrand LLP
Hartford, Connecticut

Foreword by Philip Caper, MD

Epilogue by the Honorable Bill Frist, MD
(U.S. Senator, Tennessee)

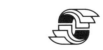

AN ASPEN PUBLICATION®
Aspen Publishers, Inc.
Gaithersburg, Maryland
1997

The authors have made every effort to ensure the accuracy of the information herein. However, appropriate information sources should be consulted, especially for new or unfamiliar procedures. It is the responsibility of every practitioner to evaluate the appropriateness of a particular opinion in the context of actual clinical situations and with due considerations to new developments. Authors, editors, and the publisher cannot be held responsible for any typographical or other errors found in this book.

Library of Congress Cataloging-in-Publication Data

The physician's guide to disease management: patient-centered care
for the 21st century / [edited by] James B. Couch
p.   cm.
Includes bibliographical references and index.
ISBN 0-8342-1003-7 (hard cover)
1. Medical protocols. 2. Outcome assessment (Medical care)
3. Medical care—Cost control. I. Couch, James B.
[DNLM: 1. Disease Management. 2. Patient-Centered Care—trends.
W 84.7 P578 1997]
RC64.P48   1997
362.1'068—dc21
DNLM/DLC
for Library of Congress
97-18244
CIP

Orders: (800) 638-8437
Customer Service: (800) 234-1660

About Aspen Publishers • For more than 35 years, Aspen has been a leading professional publisher in a variety of disciplines. Aspen's vast information resources are available in both print and electronic formats. We are committed to providing the highest quality information available in the most appropriate format for our customers. Visit Aspen's Internet site for more information resources, directories, articles, and a searchable version of Aspen's full catalog, including the most recent publications: **http://www.aspenpub.com**
Aspen Publishers, Inc. • The hallmark of quality in publishing
Member of the worldwide Wolters Kluwer group.

Editorial Resources: Brian MacDonald
Library of Congress Catalog Card Number: 97-18244
ISBN: 0-8342-1003-7

Printed in the United States of America

1 2 3 4 5

I dedicate this book to my wonderful wife, Maryann; my three great kids, John, Katherine, and Laura; and my parents, John and Betty Couch, whose command of the English language hopefully has been imparted to their son at last.

Table of Contents

Contributors

Spencer Borden IV, MD, MBA
Medical Director
Value Health Sciences
Santa Monica, California

David J. Brailer, MD, PhD
Chief Executive Officer
Care Management Science Corp
Adjunct Assistant Professor
The Wharton School
University of Pennsylvania
Clinical Associate Professor of
    Internal Medicine
University of Pennsylvania Health
    System
Philadelphia, Pennsylvania

John J. Byrnes, MD
President and CEO
Lovelace Healthcare Innovations
Vice President for Quality Improve-
    ment
Lovelace Health Systems
Albuquerque, New Mexico

Philip Caper, MD
Chief Executive Officer
Codman Research Group
Andover, Massachusetts

James B. Couch, MD, JD, FACPE
Director-in-Charge
Disease Management Consulting
Coopers & Lybrand LLP
Hartford, Connecticut

Jason Dandridge
Graduate Student, The Wharton
    School
The University of Pennsylvania
Care Management Science Corp
Philadelphia, Pennsylvania

**Tony Felton, MBBS (Hon),
    DRCOG, MRCGP, MBA**
Advisor to the Health Care and
    Pharmaceutical Group
Coopers & Lybrand
Uxbridge, Middlesex, Great Britain

Senator Bill Frist, MD
U.S. Senate
Washington, DC

Geneen Graber, PharmD
Cedars-Sinai Medical Center
Beverly Hills, California

Margaret J. Gunter, PhD
Vice President and Executive
  Director
Lovelace Clinic Foundation
Albuquerque, New Mexico

Larry L. Hipp, MD, MSc
Vice President, Managed Care
Joint Commission on Accreditation of
  Healthcare Organizations
Oakbrook Terrace, Illinois

David Levy, MD, MSc, FACPM
Chairman & CEO
Franklin Health, Inc.
Upper Saddle River, New Jersey

John Lucas, MD, MPH
President and Chief Executive Officer
Saint Francis Health System
Tulsa, Oklahoma
former Chief Executive Officer
Lovelace Health Systems
Albuquerque, New Mexico

Robert E. McCormack, MD
Associate Medical Director, Quality
  Improvement
Humana Health Care Plans
Kansas City, Missouri

Harald Rinde, MD, MBA
International Liaison Officer
Novartis Pharmaceuticals
Former Head, Global Disease
  Management
Ciba-Geigy, Ltd.
Basel, Switzerland

Scott Weingarten, MD, MPH
Director, Health Services Research
Cedars-Sinai Medical Center
Beverly Hills, California

Foreword

Philip Caper

The title of this book might give the prospective reader the impression that "disease management," "outcomes management," and "patient-centered care" are new concepts being readied for use in the 21st century. But haven't physicians always been patient centered, haven't they managed diseases (or tried to do so), and haven't they been guided by what they believe to be the best outcomes? What has changed? Is this just a new book about old subjects?

I don't think so. I believe the changes to be real and important in at least two major respects. First, as a result of the spread of managed care, a change in perspective is occurring that will change the culture of medicine for both doctors and patients in very important ways. A population-focused—that is, epidemiological—perspective of medicine has been added to the traditional patient- and doctor-focused perspectives so familiar to clinicians. Second, advances in information technology (both new analytic techniques and more powerful ways to manage and communicate data and other information) are making it possible to provide clinicians with ways of looking at medical care that have not been previously possible.

A major paradigm shift in the organization and delivery of medical care is now under way,[1] fueled by a change from fee-for-service to capitation payment for medical care benefits. That shift was initially driven by the private sector during the early 1990s but is rapidly spreading to Medicare, Medicaid, and other public sector programs.[2]

Health services research done during the past 20 years clearly documents the discretionary nature of medical care[3] with respect to *where, when,* or even *whether* particular medical services will be provided. In 1983, for example, the system of payments to hospitals was changed from one based on costs to one based on fixed prices per admission that were determined by the patient's diagnosis (diagnosis-related groups [DRGs]). Whereas cost-based reimbursement sends the message "Do whatever seems necessary—costs don't matter," DRG-based payment sends a very different message: "If what you do costs more than we'll pay, you lose money. But if you can find ways to deliver care for less, you get to keep the difference." Patterns of hospital care that had taken decades to evolve changed quickly in response to these changed financial incentives. The sensitivity of discretionary medical judgments to financial and other incentives creates powerful opportunities for management and efficiency improvement, as well as risks to the quality of care.

The paradigm shift now under way is going to make the change from cost-based reimbursement to DRGs look tame by comparison. Unlike the earlier shift (which was confined entirely to hospitals), the shift from fee-for-service to capitation payment is driving and will continue to drive major structural changes throughout the health care industry.

For a capitation payment to work, it must be administered by an organization capable of

- accepting and managing a per capita payment for a defined population
- managing and integrating a broad and complex range of services covered by that payment
- enrolling a defined population
- accepting responsibility for what happens (or does not happen) to *all* of its enrollees—not just those who happen to become patients
- managing to generate margin (whether it is called a profit does not matter) within a budget
- being sufficiently innovative and member friendly to compete with other plans for members

In fee-for-service medicine (usually coupled with indemnity insurance) potential patients are not *known* to exist until they hit the system and generate a claim. But in capitated health care delivery systems, the plan is required to know who is enrolled as well as who becomes a patient. This provides (for the first time) the opportunity to take a population-focused perspective, assessing systematically the health status and medical service use patterns of entire member populations even before they become sick enough to require care. For the first time, it may be possible to identify systematically subpopulations at risk (hypertensives, diabetics, and asthmatics, for example) early in the course of their illness in an attempt to head off avoidable progression of their disease. Much of this book is devoted to examining that topic.

Under managed care, a medical care system that has been characterized by increasing specialization and fragmentation and by little if any attention to efficiency is being brought under a management umbrella on a grand scale. It is being given strong rewards for efficiency and strong penalties for inefficiency. This development is providing an opportunity to rationalize the way medical care is delivered at the local level, within the private sector and without massive and highly centralized regulation. These are objectives that 25 years of vigorously pursued public sector initiatives have failed to accomplish.

In an unstructured fee-for-service system, micromanagement of medical care (in both public and private sectors) was the only way to control its costs. This environment spawned increasingly prescriptive regulation of the scope of insurance benefits, professional fees, institutional budgets, system capacity (implemented through certificate-of-need laws), and even individual procedures (second surgical opinions, rigidly applied protocols, preadmission, and concurrent review of hospital care). In contrast, by directly limiting per capita costs, health maintenance organizations (HMOs) and other "managed-care" systems hold the potential for drastically reducing the need for such inflexible, often rigidly applied, and always contentious techniques, which have been generally centrally directed by payers or insurance companies. The demise of centrally determined techniques of this type will free managed-care plans to innovate at the local level.

By rigidly prescribing which services will or will not be covered by fee for service, unbudgeted mechanisms of paying for medical care have locked in place dysfunctional ways of doing things (like covering some procedures in an inpatient setting but excluding them if they are performed in a less expensive outpatient setting). These restrictions have acted as a powerful deterrent to the development of efficiency-improving innovation. Only after fee-for-service modes of payment have been replaced can real progress be made.

A case in point is the On Lok program in San Francisco. For the past 20 years or so, the innovators responsible for the development of On Lok have demonstrated the power of capitated payment. In exchange for accepting the budgetary discipline of capitated payment, On Lok has been given the freedom to spend Medicare and Medicaid dollars in innovative ways. As a result, it is able to provide many additional services (such as day care, transportation, meals on wheels, and home care) to some of the most frail and high-cost elderly in their communities for no more than the cost of hospital, nursing home, and physician services in a fee-for-service environment. This model has now spread to other communities. The very structure of medical care delivery systems will demand that clinicians be concerned with and think about entire populations at risk, in addition to individual patients.

The second major change involves information technology. Advances in the manipulation, communication, and display of electronic data have made it feasible to measure the characteristics and medical care use and cost patterns for very large populations in great detail. Though most of the data being used for these purposes is currently administrative, we are rapidly moving into an era when clinical data will be available electronically, where it can be more easily analyzed and where the results can be communicated to doctors and to plan members and management. This will enable statistical process control quality improvement techniques to be applied to populations as a whole in medical care for the first time. These techniques will provide insights concerning the costs, quality, and effectiveness of medical care in ways that patient- and doctor-focused approaches alone cannot achieve.[4] For example, for the first time we are able to monitor and measure *underutilization* as well as overutilization and to track the effects of clinical or administrative innovation on the costs, quality, and outomes of care for whole populations.

This book gives the reader a quick look at some of the recent advances in the art of medical management and at some of the things that such advances, coupled with rapidly evolving information technology, can accomplish. The good news is that they are only the beginning of what medical management has the potential to achieve.

References

1. Caper P. Shifting to a new medical care paradigm. *Infocare.* 1995;2:46–50.
2. Wennberg JE, Gittlesohn A. Variations in medical care among small areas. *Sci Am.* 1982; 246:120–134.
3. Duffy S, and Forely D. Patterns of decline among inpatient procedure. *Public Health Reports.* 1996;110.
4. Caper P. The epidemiologic surveillance of medical care. *Am J Public Health.* 1987;77:669–670.

Preface

"Disease management" is an unfortunate term. Its name perpetuates the image of a sickness as opposed to a health care system. However, in this country, the former is precisely what we have had at least since 1965 (when the Medicare Law was passed), and, possibly since the 1940's when "health" insurance came into full swing.

But disease management, as developed in this book, is intended to describe a new approach to improving the health status of populations to the greatest extent per dollar invested. This is hardly the kind of pathology-focused, one-patient-at-a-time "system" that has driven this country's health care costs past the trillion dollar threshold with little systematic analysis of the payback for such a prodigious investment. In fact, many of the largest improvements in health status at a population level may be attributed to relatively cost-effective public health and environmental interventions such as water purification, immunizations, and various anti-pollution measures, among others.

This book is intended to develop disease management as a systematic population-level approach to address the age-old challenge that has finally been applied to health care: "How to get more with less?" The Foreword sets the stage for this. The first five chapters are intended to introduce disease management and its infrastructure (its knowledge base foundation, process standardization methods, outcomes measurement and data requirements, and information technology supports). The second five chapters demonstrate its application by or on behalf of key health care stakeholders (integrated delivery systems, managed care organizations, pharmaceutical firms, employers, and patients). The Epilogue takes disease management to the public policy level as a means to accommodate the twin demands of containing health care costs as a necessary concomitant of balancing the budget, while addressing the growing demands of consumers for a delivery system that is more responsive to their needs.

Although trying to coordinate the schedules of the extremely busy and talented authors of this work has been worthy of the phrase "herding cats," I have been very privileged to work with such an outstanding group. I hope that the process of editing a book, which, like legislation, may be likened to the process of producing sausage, has, nevertheless, created a product worthy of its readers.

James B. Couch

Acknowledgments

Having finished editing my first book six years ago, my usual response to any-one asking me when I would edit another was, "In my next life." Editing a book can be a very consuming task, one which I hadn't contemplated doing again, cer-tainly not, at least, during the current millennium.

So why did I do it? Like most things in life, timing was everything. Disease management (or total health management as developed in this book) has cried out for better definition and elaboration of its themes and importance. I felt very fortu-nate and privileged to have assembled an excellent group of authors and commen-tators on the subject. I believe that they have very faithfully and accurately cov-ered this emerging field. I thank them all and acknowledge their scholarship and expertise. My thanks also extend to Deb Nichols, M.D. for her outstanding contri-bution in working with Senator Frist to produce the Epilogue, despite incredible demands on both of their schedules.

But like a pebble tossed into a pond, there were many others who accommo-dated to the resulting ripples. I acknowledge both the knowledge base transfer and tremendous leeway provided to me by my friends and colleagues, Jerry Benison and Pete Solano, but especially Joe Palo, at Coopers & Lybrand. I would also like to acknowledge the tremendous talents of the entire disease management team at Coopers & Lybrand, including Steve Margolis, MD, Michele Pesanello, Carol Reynolds-Geary, Sabine Kuhn, Elisabeth Normand, and Kathy Martin, who have always made my life and work easier and more rewarding. I also acknowledge the invaluable assistance of my editorial assistant, Tracy Hains, without whom this book would still be a foot-high stack of manuscripts sitting somewhere among the debris on my desk. Most of all, I'd like to acknowledge my loving wife, Maryann, and three wonderful children, John, Katherine, and Laura, who have been the most understanding and supportive of all throughout the many hours of the past year editing this book which cut into my precious time with them. Somehow, we all got

xvii

through yet another "gestation and birthing process," successfully together. Thanks also to the outstanding child care provided by our children's loving grandmothers, Ursula Guill and Betty Couch.

Finally, I'd like to acknowledge the tremendous support and assistance from the professionals at Aspen Publishers: Brian MacDonald, Ruth Bloom, and Jennifer Barnes-Eliot, but especially Jack Bruggeman. Jack, thank you for persuading me to experience "my next life" somewhat sooner than I had anticipated.

James B. Couch

CHAPTER 1

Disease Management: An Overview

James B. Couch

ORIGINS AND EVOLUTION

Disease management (DM) is a term of art that has evolved predominantly in the managed-care and pharmaceutical industries since 1993. The term began to be used at managed-care conferences in the spring of 1993. However, it did not really take off until the pharmaceutical giant Merck & Co. bought Medco Cost Containment Services of Montvale, New Jersey, in the fall of 1993.

The DM movement accelerated in 1994 with the purchases of Diversified Pharmaceutical Services (DPS) by SmithKline Beecham and of PCS by Eli Lilly, Inc. The initial purpose of these acquisitions was to capture marketing distribution channels into managed-care organizations (MCOs). However, after having made this $13+ billion in investments, the companies realized that they could leverage these resources and contacts through them with tens of millions of patients and their providers to develop state-of-the-art programs to manage various diseases of these large populations.

Disease management has become one of the industry's most often mentioned, yet least understood buzzwords during the 1993 to 1997 time period. There have been books published on it (including this one). There have been newsletters (eg, *Disease State Management*, by American Health Consultants). There have been dozens of conferences and seminars, including five very well attended "Disease Management Congresses" sponsored by the most successful managed-care conference organization in the world, the National Managed Health Care Congress. Even more significantly, individuals, units, sections, divisions, departments, and even whole companies have been using the term in their titles.

Many other organizations have made major financial, technological, and human resource commitments to DM, including (but not limited to)

- *Managed-care organizations,* such as United Health Care, Harvard Pilgrim Health Care, U.S. Health Care, and Group Health Cooperative of Puget Sound

- *Pharmaceutical firms,* such as Merck, SmithKline, Eli Lilly, Novartis, Glaxo, Zeneca, and Bristol Myers Squibb

- *Integrated delivery systems/group practices,* such as Henry Ford Health System, Lovelace Health System, Mayo Clinic, and Park Nicollet

- *Specialty centers,* such as National Jewish Center of Immunology and Respiratory Diseases, M. D. Anderson, and Memorial Sloan Kettering

- *Specialty organizations,* such as Value Health, Salick Health Care, U.S. Behavioral Health, and Diabetes Treatment Centers of America

- *Academic health centers/systems,* such as University of Pennsylvania Health System, Johns Hopkins Health System, and Cedars-Sinai Health System

- *Blue Cross/Blue Shield organizations,* such as Blue Cross/Blue Shield of Minnesota, Blue Cross/Blue Shield of South Carolina, Trigon (Blue Cross/ Blue Shield of Virginia), Blue Cross/Blue Shield of Missouri, and Blue Cross/Blue Shield of Florida

- *Indemnity insurers,* such as Aetna, Prudential, CIGNA, New York Life, Principal, and Mutual of Omaha

- *Professional associations,* such as Pharmaceutical Research and Manufacturers Associations (PhRMA), Association of American Health Plans (AAHP), Medical Group Management Association (MGMA), and American Group Practice Association (AGPA)

- *Multihospital chains,* such as Intermountain Health Care, Columbia HCA, and Tenet

- *Group purchasing organizations,* such as Voluntary Hospital of America (VHA), American Health Care Systems (AmHS), and Premier Health

- *Medical device companies,* such as Baxter Health Care Corporation, U.S. Surgical, and Ethicon (Johnson & Johnson)

- *Employers and coalitions,* such as Xerox, GTE, Digital, Central Florida Health Care Coalition, Memphis Business Group on Health, Midwest Business Group on Health, and Business Health Care Action Group (BHCAG)

- *Pharmaceutical benefit companies,* such as Medco, PCS, DPS, Value Rx, and Caremark

- *"Independent" disease management companies,* such as Stuart Disease Management, and Greenstone Health Care

It should be clear from the above that there is tremendous interest in DM as a strategy for improving the demonstrable quality and cost-effectiveness of health care delivery. But what is DM and what is (or should be) its role in improving health care delivery?

DEFINITION

To paraphrase Forrest Gump, "Disease management is as disease management does." The term *disease management* has acquired many definitions in the past few years, depending on the context in which it is used. When it is used in the context of capitated managed care and other prospectively financial arrangements, it has been regarded as a concept or methodology to permit providers and/or payers to assume varying degrees of risk for the costs of treating a population through standardizing the care of patients within defined disease groups. The emphasis there is on identifying patients possessing specific diseases and then developing therapeutic programs with the greatest probability for good clinical outcomes at acceptable cost levels, based on the best evidence in the medical literature, clinical databases, and other sources. DM thus permits capitated managed-care groups and other prospectively financed health care organizations to stay within their allocated financial resources. If possible, they may generate a profit even as it can be documented that patients' clinical outcomes, quality of life, and satisfaction improve.

A subset to this operational definition of DM would involve the perspective of pharmaceutical firms (see Chapter 8). Pharmaceutical and medical device firms have become very interested and involved in DM because it provides them with an opportunity to demonstrate how appropriately selected and administered drug and device interventions in various disease states may result in optimal clinical outcomes with relatively low resource consumption. These firms are especially interested in showing providers, payers, purchasers, patients, and policy makers that their agents may decrease hospitalization and emergency department (ED) admission rates, physician office visits, and other more costly interventions in consistently measurable ways. To these firms, DM may represent an avenue for documenting that *increased* use of their products and/or services may actually *decrease* the overall costs of treating patient populations with chronic diseases (eg, asthma/chronic obstructive pulmonary disease, diabetes, congestive heart failure, arthritis/low back pain, gastrointestinal problems) while improving clinical outcomes and stakeholder satisfaction.

Practitioners (especially physicians) often regard DM quizzically. They are convinced that they have been "doing DM" since they laid hands on their first patient. In some sense, they are right. However, in the broad sense, most practitioners have been practicing medicine (or otherwise delivering health care) that is based only on their own experience (or perhaps on the experience of their group or organization).

Many physicians and other practitioners at world-famous health care organizations who have been managing their patients with various diseases on the basis of institutional norms have not been practicing disease management as it is defined and developed in this chapter and throughout this book. Adhering to a prestigious organization's experience and norms for treating patients (though admirable) may still be too provincial or (as discussed later) more practitioner-biased than patient-centered (see Chapter 10).

Purchasers, payers, and policy makers also have their own perspectives on what DM should be or should do (see the section "Stakeholder Needs" below). Needless to say, their overriding goal for DM is to provide a more rational, systematic, and ultimately more efficient and cost-effective way to diagnose and treat patient populations, the costs of whose care they either subsidize or underwrite in the private or public sector.

Some of the more progressive of these stakeholders are beginning to realize that putting quality first is ultimately the most cost-effective approach. Some (especially major manufacturers such as GM, Ford, Motorola, Xerox, Digital, and GTE; see Chapter 9) have begun to apply to health benefits the total quality management, process redesign, and time-based management methods (among others) that have dramatically improved their product development and manufacturing processes. For them, disease management has provided a methodology for extending these tried and true industrial management methods to the important area of extracting optimal value from their health plans and the practitioners serving their work force.

Given these various perspectives, can there be a working definition of DM? For purposes of this chapter and book, DM will be defined as *a knowledge-based process intended to improve continuously the value of health care delivery from the perspectives of those who receive, purchase, provide, supply, and evaluate it.* This working definition is intended to be fairly comprehensive in its scope. It is intended to encompass the whole notion of "value" in health care—that is, optimal clinical, economic, quality-of-life, and satisfaction outcomes for the lowest possible expenditure of resources, time, and "hassles."

HEALTH CARE VALUE

Health care value can be defined by the following equation·

$$\text{Health Care Value} = \frac{\text{Quality of Clinical, Economic, Service, and Humanistic Outcomes}}{\text{Overall Costs, Time, Resources, and "Hassles"}}$$
$$\text{to All Stakeholders}$$

This component of the DM definition may be dissected down much further depending on the particular nature of the DM initiative. First, the definition of health care value must apply to the specific disease(s), illness(es), or condition(s) targeted to be managed more cost-effectively. Outcomes that must be further delineated may include (but not be limited to)

- Objective clinical outcomes
    1. mortality rates
    2. morbidity rates
    3. complication rates
    4. infection rates
    5. hospitalization rates
    6. ED admission rates

- Subjective outcomes (perception and satisfaction)
    1. patient perceptions of care
    2. patient and provider satisfaction
    3. willingness to recommend care
    4. health plan reenrollment rates

- Humanistic and quality-of-life outcomes (please refer to the SF-36 and SF-12 or the New England Medical Center and Health Outcomes Institute of Stratis Health)
    1. physical functioning
    2. role functioning (as a parent, spouse, worker, etc)
    3. social functioning
    4. pain levels
    5. energy levels
    6. fatigue levels
    7. mental well-being
    8. overall perception of health status

- Economic outcomes
    1. overall hospital costs/time period saved
    2. overall ED costs/time period saved
    3. overall outpatient costs/time period saved
    4. physician-related costs/time period saved

5. pharmaceutical-related costs/time period saved
6. procedural costs/time period saved
7. laboratory costs/time period saved
8. overall health costs/time period (across the spectrum of care) saved
9. per-member per-month (year) costs for all of the above saved

The denominator of the health care value equation represents the algebraic sum total of the costs in time, resources, and "hassles" involved in health care delivery from the perspectives of those who provide, purchase, receive, or evaluate it. Quantifying this denominator requires an additional breakdown of its components. For example, on the provider end, the "costing" of specific interventions involves the financial quantification of the direct and indirect labor and materials costs involved in designing, developing, and delivering those interventions intended to achieve optimal improvements in the various outcomes of targeted subpopulations.

As the saying goes, "Time is money." This lesson has certainly been learned in industries other than health care. As stated earlier (and elaborated more in Chapter 9), many of the most progressive corporations are applying the latest management methodologies to the important health benefits management arena. Turnaround time has become an important outcome indicator of quality in both manufacturing and service-based businesses. It is increasingly being applied as a measurement of health care quality. In the future, patients (and their health care sponsors) will evaluate health care organizations on their ability not only to improve the health status of populations in measurable ways but also to do it faster to minimize absenteeism and other productivity losses.

Finally, there is the "hassle" component. Although there may not currently be a standardized "hasslemeter," this is a very real concern of all stakeholders (especially physicians and patients). Much of the "hassle" component can probably be minimized by optimizing all the other components of the health care value equation. However, the "hassle factor" (or the anticipation of its effects by stakeholders) may well constitute the largest single impediment to the delivery of optimal health care. Therefore, any well-designed and implemented disease management intervention must address and minimize this potential "showstopper" right from the start.

WHAT DM IS NOT (OR SHOULD NOT BE)

We can further clarify the definition of DM by indicating what it is not (or should not be). DM is not (or should not be)

- a marketing ploy to get certain drugs on health plans' formularies
- value-added pharmaceutical marketing ("turbo-marketing")

- self-serving "outcomes research" (i.e., to "prove" that one's plan or drug or device or process is better than that of competitors)
- disease-focused "carve-outs"

Unfortunately, DM has become too strongly associated with various programmatic methods for pharmaceutical firms to improve their marketing to managed care and integrated delivery systems. Thus, many have come to regard it cynically as the latest marketing buzzword that pharmaceutical firms are using to ingratiate themselves to health plans and employers encountering significant costs in the treatment of patient groups with specific diseases.

However, DM needs to transcend marketing, and even research and development and clinical affairs, to realize its full potential. DM is not a mechanism to "carve out" specific diseases as part of a capitated-payment arrangement. DM in its pure sense is population-based medicine (see the foreword to this book). DM recognizes that individuals and, even more, populations cannot be neatly categorized (or "carved out") into specific disease groups. Good DM requires a systematic process for identifying, evaluating, diagnosing, and treating populations of patients on the basis of best evidence from controlled clinical trials and outcomes knowledge bases to produce the greatest achievable improvements in collective health status per interventional dollar invested.

WHY DM IS SO IMPORTANT NOW

As we approach the next millennium, an unprecedented alignment of forces and incentives is occurring across the public and private sectors in this and other countries around the world. The ascendancy of DM can be traced all the way back to the global telecommunications revolution and the cascade of effects that it has had on all human endeavors, especially such a deeply personal, yet information-driven service as health care. The worldwide telecommunications revolution, especially in Internet and Intranet technologies, is rapidly transforming the way that many of us receive and provide information. This is unleashing a consumer revolution of enormous proportions that is dramatically increasing global competition for all products and services. The marketplace is now the world. With all the consumer debt out there and the desire for ever-increasing levels of quality, the demand for demonstrable value far outstrips any sense of company (or even country) loyalty in this new global marketplace.

Because of this demand for value in all products and services, not only companies but countries around the world are reexamining the way they do business, including the way they evaluate and manage their own suppliers of products and services. In the past few years, both companies and countries have recognized that their largest and perhaps most important suppliers are those providing health care products and services. Hence, at the same time that Internet and Intranet technologies have forced companies to improve the demonstrable value of their products and services, these same companies are using their advanced technologies to assess the value of the health benefits that their employees and families are receiving.

The most progressive companies (regardless of national origins) are recognizing how much their overall productivity (and profitability) is dependent on having healthy employees with healthy families who are satisfied with their jobs and benefits (especially health insurance). Minimizing absenteeism, long- and short-term disability costs, and productivity losses has become a major goal of these forward-thinking companies. Achieving these goals requires the right kinds of relationships with the right kinds of health plans and providers.

These companies must engage in supplier value management, and, more specifically, health care value management, to channel their employees and families into the health plans with the best track record for achieving work force health status improvement goals. To ensure this, they (as well as public sector purchasers) are entering into partnerships with like-minded health plans and provider systems to collect, share, and evaluate the necessary performance data for demonstrating linkages between certain health practices and clinical interventions and the achievement of these business goals.

To achieve these goals for their purchaser customers' health plans, provider groups and their suppliers are conceiving, designing, developing, and implementing DM programs as defined in this chapter. These programs represent "in-the-trenches" methods to achieve the health benefits goals of their purchaser customers. Their customers, in turn, recognize that they must achieve these goals if they are to put out the best possible products and services to *their* customers in the global marketplace. This cascade of forces driving DM is depicted in Figure 1–1.

THE DM PROCESS

If DM is regarded as a project or a program, it will be the first thing eliminated during a time of fiscal belt tightening at any type of health care organization. But DM is a process. Rather than being just another business process, it is a transformational process intended to change fundamentally the way that any type of health care organization regards itself and its customers, employees, and suppliers. DM provides a new way of aligning the inputs and outputs of customers and suppliers up and down the value chain that ultimately results in demonstrably better value care to patients and those who subsidize overall costs of care. In that respect, it is not a process that can be pigeonholed into any one department, division, or even subsidiary of an organization. Rather, it must serve to link the diverse

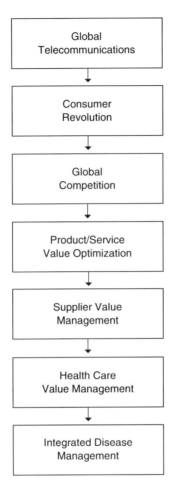

Figure 1–1 Forces Driving the Ascendancy of Disease Management. Courtesy of Coopers & Lybrand, Hartford, Connecticut.

disciplines that need to be brought together to serve the needs of the ultimate customer (the patient) better (Figure 1–2).

DM needs to be regarded as a mobilizing and unifying process within a health care organization. It may be regarded as a strategy. However, in a larger sense, as the voice of the customer, it should drive the strategy of better meeting the needs of a stakeholder-driven marketplace. In this way, marketing may focus the

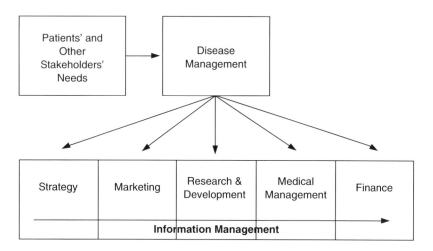

Figure 1–2 Disease Management Unifies Diverse Disciplines To Serve the Patient. Courtesy of Coopers & Lybrand, Hartford, Connecticut.

organization's efforts within those strategic parameters. This, in turn, will provide a road map for research and development to design and ultimately to deliver the products and services that are and will be demanded by the marketplace. Medical management may then allocate its clinical resources to support best the delivery of the organization's products and services in the marketplace. Finally, finance can provide the human, technological, and monetary resources necessary to achieve business goals and objectives with optimal operational efficiencies. This will minimize the waste that occurs so often in organizations that do not unify their component parts in this stakeholder-driven strategy.

But even transformational processes like DM need to have process steps. DM may be regarded as a series of steps that are ultimately part of a continuous value improvement process that should drive any organization (especially a health care organization). These steps are shown in Figure 1–3 and discussed below.

Knowledge Base Creation

DM, as a process driving progressive health care organizations, must begin, as depicted in Figure 1–2, with the patient (or, more accurately, with the identified needs of a population of patients, the costs of whose care are underwritten by either private or public sector purchasers). Identifying their needs, as well as the needs of those who subsidize their care, is the first step in creating a *stakeholder*

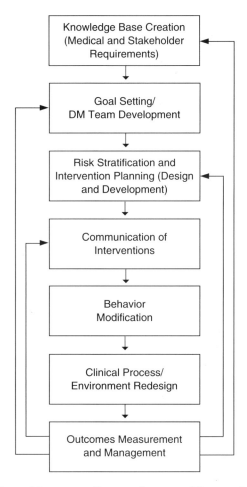

Figure 1–3 The Disease Management Process. Courtesy of Coopers & Lybrand, Hartford, Connecticut.

---

requirements knowledge base that will drive the remaining steps of the DM process.

The other component of the knowledge base, the *medical requirements knowledge base,* consists of the best scientific evidence (from controlled clinical studies, the medical literature, outcomes-validated databases, and other sources) concerning which clinical processes have achieved the best results in populations of patients with particular diseases for the least expenditure of resources (see Chapters

2, 3, and 4). The term *evidence-based medicine* has increasingly been applied to this undertaking. But creation and usage of the medical knowledge base are insufficient if this knowledge base is not coupled to the stakeholder requirements knowledge base discussed above. In fact, the stakeholder requirements knowledge base in DM as defined here will drive (or at least shape) how the medical knowledge base is created. The medical knowledge base created should reflect the best evidence concerning which diagnostic and therapeutic processes are most likely to achieve the outcomes set by the stakeholders (within realistic limits). The interplay of these two components produces the actual knowledge base that drives the rest of the DM process.

Goal Setting and Team Development

The next step of the DM process concerns establishing realistic goals or outcomes of the DM process, based on stakeholder requirements and the best evidence about what may be possible to achieve. It is at this point that very specific outcome measurement indicators should be established and validated with the stakeholders.

Once these goals are set, the other part of this step involves formation of an appropriate cross-disciplinary team composed of professionals with the most in-depth knowledge of the steps of the specific DM process targeted for improvement. Depending on the particular DM process, team members may include (but not be limited to)

- *Physicians,* including specialists and subspecialists with a disease-specific subject matter expertise and clinical experience
- *Nurses,* also with disease-specific subject matter expertise and practice experience
- *Pharmacists or doctors of pharmacology* with in-depth expertise and experience with the alternative therapeutic agents for the particular disease state
- *Marketers* with expertise concerning the relative acceptance and usage, among practitioners, of these alternative therapeutic agents
- *Financial and actuarial professionals* familiar with cost-benefit analyses who may work with the clinical experts to evaluate the feasibility and probable return on investment of alternative interventions (including whether those interventions can be cost justified with capitation and other risk-sharing arrangements)
- *Statistical experts* who can help structure disease management pilot projects likely to demonstrate significant improvements at least following (if not actually caused by) specific interventions

• *Communication experts* who can translate technical interventions into patient-friendly language and formats with the greatest likelihood of changing behavior

Having the appropriate team assembled to achieve realistic and measurable goals (outcomes driven by the stakeholder requirements and medical knowledge base) permits the creation of interventions that can most likely be implemented to achieve the intended results.

Risk Stratification and Intervention Planning

The next step in the DM process may involve *practice guideline development, intervention design and development,* and/or *practice standardization.* The common denominator is that populations and subpopulations of patients have been identified for whom the best medical evidence would indicate that specific types of interventions will probably result in the most desirable outcomes (from the various stakeholders' perspectives).

An important component of this process step is risk or illness/condition severity stratification (see Chapter 4). By whatever name, interventions, clinical guidelines, or practice standardization must be specific to populations and subpopulations with roughly comparable illness/condition severities, risk factors, and probabilities for certain outcomes (clinical, financial, and humanistic). This is required for at least the following reasons:

• Patients must be grouped into comparable illness categories so that appropriately intensive interventions can be designed.
• Illness categories permit the strata-specific cost-benefit analyses necessary to allocate intervention resources most cost-effectively.
• Clinical, financial, and quality-of-life measurements are most appropriately applied to patients falling into specific risk strata (e.g., mortality rates or even hospitalization days per 1000 days would not be appropriate measurement indicators for the least sick individuals of a population afflicted with practically any type of disease).
• An identification of the risk factors driving patients into various strata is necessary for design of specific interventions with the greatest likelihood of optimal impact on patients' outcomes.

It is important that whatever risk stratification method is used, there be some method for evaluating its accuracy in classifying patients into the appropriate intervention groups. This is important because falsely stratifying patients may have quite significant medical, economic, and legal consequences.

Assuming that there is a validated risk stratification method, interventions may be designed to address the specific pathology or behaviors responsible for the increased likelihood of undesirable clinical, financial, and/or quality-of-life outcomes. Practice then may be standardized around those clinical processes that have the greatest probability of achieving these desired outcomes as supported by the scientific and statistical literature.

Communication of Interventions

The next step of the DM process is communicating the interventions, guidelines, or standardized practices to both practitioners and patients in a manner most likely to change their preintervention clinical decision making. The importance of this process step is often underrated, perhaps because it is regarded as more of an art than the other steps. However, without its successful execution, everything completed before and after it will be for naught.

The most important variables in this step are the message content, the media for delivery, and the feedback. Even the most rigorously validated, evidence-based guidelines must be recast into appropriate language to influence the clinical decision-making behavior of practitioners as well as patients (see Chapters 3 and 10). To accomplish this may require some or all of the following:

- input from practitioners and patients concerning the content of the intervention
- surveys or focus groups of practitioners or patients to react to both the message and the media
- comparisons of various media or formats concerning their effectiveness (eg, spoken, written, electronic)
- postimplementation feedback evaluation of the effectiveness of various communication methods in actually changing the clinical decision making of practitioners and patients

Behavior Modification

The next step of the process concerns behavior modification. This step is tightly linked to the immediately previous step. In fact, it is the goal of this previous step. However, true behavior modification may well require more than even the best communication of well-validated interventions. Behaviors of both practitioners and patients may be very much ingrained. All of us as patients (or potential patients) may be able to recite line and verse the path to optimal health. We may well be convinced of the evidence supporting the need to stop smoking, limit alcohol intake, maintain body weight within an acceptable range, eat a low-fat and high-fiber diet, avoid undue stress, exercise regularly, and floss daily. None of that means, however, that we are going to follow all (or even most) of these guidelines on a regular basis, despite the strong evidence that doing so would enhance both our longevity and our quality of life.

This also applies to many practitioners who just will not use angiotensin converting enzyme (ACE) inhibitors for their heart failure patients, or who refuse to use steroid inhalants in their severe asthmatics, or who believe that a drug-treatable bacterium (*Helicobacter pylori*) could not possibly cause ulcers. Medicine has a long tradition of individualistic physicians who base their clinical decision-making behavior on the grounds of their own experience and not the collective wisdom.

An evaluation of various behavior modification methods is beyond the scope of this chapter. The relative success that different organizations have had in changing at least practitioners' behavior is discussed in Chapters 3, 6, 7, and 10. As with life in general, timing is everything, whether in changing practitioners' or patients' behavior. Both practitioners and patients must be convinced that the consequences of continuing with current behaviors are likely to be sufficiently bad to themselves or those close to them to justify what they may perceive as a tremendous investment of energy to change long-standing habits.

Clinical Process Redesign

The next step of the DM process, clinical process redesign, assumes that both practitioners and patients (and often other stakeholders), for whatever reason, have become predisposed to alter their clinical and lifestyle decision-making behavior. Once they are so predisposed, the "usual and customary" clinical processes need to be redesigned to accommodate and reinforce these new behaviors. Not permanently changing the environment for making these clinical decisions (including incentives, reinforcing feedback, and other influencing factors) will probably doom these new desirable behaviors to extinction.

Practitioners who do start treating their heart failure patients with ACE inhibitors, their severe asthmatic patients with steroid inhalants, or their H_2 antagonist–resistant patients with anti–*H. pylori* agents must have these new behaviors reinforced, lest there be backsliding into the old ingrained ways. DM interventions should enable various technologies to provide feedback on positive results of these behavior changes as quickly and often as possible. This feedback may need to be supplemented by various changes in the whole clinical decision support process for treating such patients to make reversion to old patterns quite difficult.

This step is especially important for patients whose new behavior may be highly fragile without the creation of a strong, reinforcing environment. Many addictive behaviors are linked. It may be very difficult for many patients to stay away from cigarettes, excess alcohol, drugs, fatty foods, or other temptations without some type of intensive stress reduction intervention. The obsession with body shape in our society may be reason enough for patients to engage in the much more deleterious habit of smoking.

To the extent possible, patients who are trying to change certain behaviors should not return to environments likely to reinforce the old behaviors. A recovering alcoholic should probably not return to his job as a bartender. Someone trying to lose weight should consider work outside a restaurant or pastry shop. Every effort should be made to provide the tools and support that patients will need to sustain the very difficult behavioral changes that they have made.

Outcomes Measurement and Management

The next step of the DM process, outcomes measurement and management, validates or invalidates the overall effectiveness of the entire DM process in terms of meeting the goals for the process established at the outset. For much more detail on this step, see Chapter 4, as well as the "real-world" results documented in Chapter 6.

Outcomes measurement assesses whether changes in behavior, clinical decision making, and other processes have produced the results set previously as stakeholder-driven goals. To measure clinical, economic, or quality-of-life outcomes, the following are necessary:

- postintervention collection of clinical, economic, and quality-of-life data on the population(s) of patients who were subject to the intervention(s) or who acted as a "control" group (who had also had such data collected on them or from them before the intervention)
- aggregation and analysis of that data
- discernment of statistically significant improvements (or at least the beginnings of favorable trends) relative to preintervention levels

An exhaustive summary of the types of data that may be collected to measure outcomes is beyond the scope of this chapter (see Chapter 4, 6, and others for more detail). However, some categories of outcomes data were referred to in the earlier section on "Health Care Value."

Sometimes, improvements in certain clinical process rates believed or proven to be associated with improved outcomes may be the goal of DM processes. These process rates may include

- medication compliance rates
- dietary compliance rates

- exercise regimen compliance rates
- practice guideline compliance rates
- vaccination compliance rates
- mammography screening compliance rates
- colorectal screening compliance rates
- diabetic retinopathy screening compliance rates
- glycosylated hemoglobin checking rates
- steroid inhalant utilization rates in severe asthmatics
- ACE inhibitor utilization rates in heart failure patients

The second component of this final step of the DM process is outcomes management (or outcomes improvement). This step compares the postintervention actual outcomes measured with those originally set as goals to be achieved through the DM process. If goals are met or exceeded, then the overall DM process is fortified so that the gains may be "locked in" and sustained. If goals are not met, the following iterative process begins:

1. Results are fed back into the knowledge base.
2. Goals are reassessed to determine how realistic they were in light of the actual results achieved.
3. The interventions (including any practice guidelines or other initiatives to standardize practice based on the best medical evidence) may need to be revised/improved.
4. The message, media, or feedback to practitioners, patients, or others of the guidelines or interventions may not be sufficiently effective and may need to be revised/improved.
5. Various other steps or components of the DM process may need to be revised/improved.
6. The whole process may need to be revised/improved.

All of the above options fall into the category of continuous quality improvement (CQI). What is important here is that these CQI processes be established and maintained. Health care organizations of whatever type engaged in the DM process that can cycle through this CQI process more quickly and effectively will succeed in the emerging value-driven health care marketplace.

STAKEHOLDER NEEDS FROM DISEASE MANAGEMENT

The first part of this chapter touched upon the notion that there are various stakeholders with a vested interest in the structure, process, and outcomes of the DM process. These stakeholders may be defined as the "seven Ps":

1. purchasers
2. payers
3. providers
4. practitioners
5. policy makers
6. product producers
7. patients

The immediately previous section stated that these stakeholders' needs and requirements for the DM process were at least as important in shaping the process as the state-of-the-art medical evidence concerning the diagnosis and treatment of various targeted diseases. More specifically, the needs (or goals) of the "seven Ps" stakeholders in relation to the DM process may be outlined as the following:

- Policy makers (government and other public sector purchasers, legislators, health policy analysts, etc)
    1. Manage overall health costs such as those from the Medicare and Medicaid programs.
    2. Improve, or at least not sacrifice, quality of care.
    3. Function in more of a managed-care environment.
    4. Demonstrate to taxpayers that value has been received/provided.

- Purchasers (employers and business coalitions)
    1. Manage overall health costs.
    2. Improve patient outcomes and employee health, productivity, and satisfaction.
    3. Prosper in a managed, perhaps capitated, health care environment.
    4. Demonstrate a favorable health benefits return on investment (ROI) to senior management and shareholders.

- Payers (insurers and managed-care organizations)
    1. Decrease per-member per-month costs.
    2. Stay within capitation allowances.
    3. Improve members' health status and plan satisfaction.
    4. Maintain and increase plan enrollment and reenrollment.
    5. Keep premiums at a competitive level.
    6. Demonstrate superior value to purchasers.

- Providers (including hospitals, health systems, long- and short-term care facilities, etc)
    1. Decrease resource utilization.
    2. Accelerate patient disclosure.

3. Decrease readmission.
4. Rationalize diagnosis and treatment.
5. Improve inpatient and outpatient outcomes.
6. Smooth transition across the spectrum of care settings.
7. Demonstrate superior value to purchasers and payers.

- Practitioners (group practices, physician organizations, practice management organizations, physicians, nurses, alternative practitioners, etc)
  1. Decrease health care utilization where cost reimbursement is capitated.
  2. Rationalize and standardize diagnosis and treatment.
  3. Improve patient outcomes.
  4. Demonstrate superior value to purchasers, payers, and patients.

- Product producers
  1. Improve product and process efficiency.
  2. Stay within capitated allowances in risk-sharing arrangements.
  3. Demonstrate superior value of products and services.
  4. Establish long-term customer relationships/partnerships.
  5. Access emerging markets.

- Patients
  1. Maintain or improve health status and productivity.
  2. Decrease health care utilization and out-of-pocket costs.
  3. Simplify and improve the effectiveness of self-care.
  4. Emphasize prevention.
  5. Improve quality of life and functioning ability.

ROLE OF DM IN THE BROADER HEALTH CARE INDUSTRY: HEALTH CARE VALUE PURCHASING

DM, as defined and developed in this book, is intended to transcend any one component of the health care industry (eg, pharmaceuticals, managed care). It should be regarded, rather, as a change in mind-set among all health care stakeholders concerning the delivery, financing, and purchasing of care.

DM is a natural outgrowth of health or medical care value purchasing. Health care value purchasing applies the same principles and practices to purchasing health benefits that both private and public entities apply to the procurement of any other product or service. This was mentioned earlier in this chapter and is discussed more in Chapter 9. However, it is instructive to see how this new corporate philosophy that applies to all forms of procurement has set the stage for DM as developed in this book.

When either a public or private sector corporate purchaser engages in value purchasing of any product or service, it undertakes a very systematic process of matching competing vendors' performance parameters against certain standards and each other. The goal of this comparative analysis is to determine which vendor comes closest to meeting the buyer's requirements at a price that, if not the lowest among competing bidders, may be justified as more expensive by the incremental *value* of the product or service from the perspective of the purchaser. Thus, value purchasing does not necessarily favor the lowest bidder, unless the lowest bidder can also demonstrate superior quality in meeting and exceeding the buyer's requirements.

In the health care industry, the practice of value purchasing is finally starting to take hold and should intensify in the near future as efforts to contain costs, balance budgets, eliminate deficits, and preserve quality accelerate. In America, there has been a significant backlash against managed care in the past year or two. Much of this has arisen from such controversial developments as "gag clauses" that prohibit physicians from informing patients of various treatment options not accepted by particular health plans. Lately, however, there has been a growing sentiment that managed care in general may compromise quality on the altar of cost savings. "Drive-through" deliveries and mastectomies have become major sources of criticism.

That is where health care value purchasing practiced by major private and public sector buyers may play an important role to ensure that quality is preserved (but at a reasonable cost). Value purchasing of health care focuses on the entire package of health care services delivered to a covered population in a specific time period. It also accounts for the satisfaction of individual patients with health plans, systems, and providers. How well a health plan or other system of providers can demonstrate that it meets both macro and micro requirements will determine its success in gaining access to patient populations in the future era of health care value purchasing.

Given such a world of health care value purchasing, DM provides the road map to success. DM is a methodology for translating purchasers' population-based (macro) and patient-centered (micro) requirements into criteria and standards that providers and suppliers must meet to gain access to the population of patients that these large purchasers control.

TOTAL HEALTH MANAGEMENT

To the extent that DM can work to standardize treatment around certain guidelines or other clinical processes for specific conditions, it may rightly be called *disease management*. However, when DM aspires to the higher calling of providing a means for both purchasers and providers to optimize the demonstrable value of health care delivery to a large population of patients with a wide variety of diseases and conditions of varying severity, it may more accurately be defined as total health management (THM).

In the next 3 to 5 years, DM will either evolve into THM or slowly fade away from the health care lexicon. Those organizations, especially pharmaceutical firms, that expected DM to increase sales and profitability in the relatively short term are now reconsidering their commitment to DM (see Chapter 8). The problem is that they were not really committed to DM in the first place, at least not in the THM sense as developed in this book. That is why those organizations that "committed" to DM in the more narrow sense have become disillusioned now. They were not as interested in making the long-term investment necessary to transform the delivery of health care products and services as they were interested in making short-term profits.

Organizations that embrace DM as the route to patient-centered care, however (see Chapter 10), have been willing to forego short-term profits in favor of making long-term investments and commitments to serving all stakeholders better. These organizations recognize that the purchasers of their products and services in the next century will be dramatically different from those of the recent past. They recognize that the focus is to demonstrate the delivery of superior-value products and services to covered populations, while satisfying the needs of individual patients and their families. This constitutes the management of the total health (preventive and public health, early detection, diagnosis, treatment and ongoing monitoring) of covered populations (ie, THM).

To be effective, DM as THM must truly be knowledge based and patient centered, as discussed earlier and in Chapters 2, 3, 4, 5, and 10 of this book. Each population's health needs must be thoroughly dissected, sliced and diced, aggregated and disaggregated, analyzed and reanalyzed so that the allocation of resources is not only most appropriate but optimally effective and efficient. Any organization committed to succeeding in DM as THM must accept and commit to what will truly be a new and different (and often daunting) way of doing business. It will need to make tremendous investments in information technology, medical management, human resources, behavioral management, and alliance management to succeed (Figure 1–4).

In Figure 1–4, DM as THM may be represented by all the areas covered by the interlocking circles. All these areas relate to any organization in the business of managing the total health of covered populations. There are, however, certain areas (not necessarily drawn to specific scale or location) where no one health care organization can undertake DM as THM alone. These "gaps" may appear in any (and usually appear in all) of the three overlapping circles of competency: (1) medical management of populations, (2) information management, and (3) behavioral management.

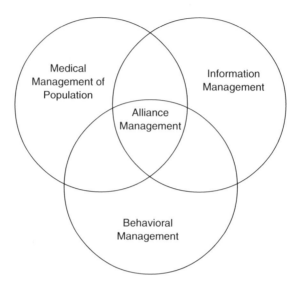

Figure 1–4 Disease Management as Total Health Management. Courtesy of Coopers & Lybrand, Hartford, Connecticut.

It is where these gaps appear that a fourth component of DM as THM may complete the puzzle. This is the component of alliance management. Alliance management as a distinct discipline for completing the puzzle for organizations engaged in DM as THM is covered in the next section of this chapter.

ALLIANCE MANAGEMENT TO COMPLETE THE PUZZLE

If any one phenomenon has dramatically distinguished the 1990s global business world, it is the explosive growth of strategic alliances. Major pharmaceutical firms are getting together (eg, Ciba and Sandoz, Pharmacia and Upjohn, Glaxo and Burroughs Wellcome), as are telecommunication firms and cable companies (eg, British Telecom and MCI), major health care providers and managed-care companies (eg, Columbia HCA Health Care Corporation and Value Health), software companies and network television (Microsoft and the National Broadcasting Company, MSNBC), and major multimedia entertainment companies and international publishing and newscast organizations (Time Warner).

As depicted in Figure 1–4, DM as THM is a perfect candidate for the special breed of strategic alliances starting to emerge in the trillion-dollar health care industry. What has distinguished alliances, in general, especially in the late 1990s, has been the focus on complementing markets and core competencies, not just leveraging short-term profits through the speculative takeovers, arbitrage, and other financial devices rampant in the 1980s. For these alliances to be worth their tremendous financial and emotional expense, however, they must be very carefully planned and executed.

Strategic alliances usually proceed through a series of phases not unlike those characteristic of mating rituals. These phases may include

- attraction
- approach
- exchange
- dating
- discussion
- disillusionment
- disengagement or more discussion
- engagement (possibly including prenuptial agreements)
- marriage
- eventual termination or premature divorce

Taking this analogy one step forward, organizations (from any industry) that want to pass through these phases in the most effective and least acrimonious manner should insert a crucial planning step at the very beginning: self-assessment. As so often happens in more conventional mating rituals, people often do not find the right partner for themselves because they never really understood themselves and their needs and competencies before commencing the "hunt." The next few paragraphs outline a methodology for undertaking this initial self-assessment that should permit passage through the remaining steps of alliance building more predictably and perhaps even enjoyably. The case study below represents an actual example of two leading organizations coming together that might not have ever done so in the absence of undertaking prior self-assessments.

A CASE STUDY IN ALLIANCE MANAGEMENT

A large global pharmaceutical firm and a leading integrated delivery system had been two (very large) ships passing in the night for years. The leading integrated delivery system had merely regarded the pharmaceutical firm as one of a dozen or more vendors (suitors) with nothing much in particular distinguishing itself.

The major pharmaceutical firm concluded that it needed to raise its profile from that of a vendor to the pharmacy department to that of a strategic ally at the senior executive level. The firm accomplished this by using a standardized instrument to evaluate both its own and the leading integrated delivery system's preparedness to engage in DM as THM.

Performing this standardized assessment clearly distinguished the pharmaceutical firm. Doing so created a sense of commonality, a singularity of purpose to serve patients better, and a mutual understanding of how the two organizations could join forces for optimal impact in the marketplace. Assessing each other's relative strengths and areas for improvement provided a road map for the two to engage in joint planning and ultimately to implement activities to capitalize on key components of DM as THM (see Figure 1–4).

A POSSIBLE FUTURE COURSE FOR DISEASE MANAGEMENT

Current Trends

DM is likely to evolve to the extent that leaders are committed to it as a long-term solution to extracting optimal value from the health care delivery process, as opposed to a short-term route to improved sales. Some encouraging current and probable future trends should nudge DM's evolution more toward the first scenario (see also U.S. Senator Bill Frist's epilogue to this book).

The current trend is a movement toward giving patients more power to guide their own clinical decision making. Patients and their families are wanting and demanding more user-friendly information concerning various diagnostic and therapeutic options (especially involving nonprescription drugs, self-diagnosis and treatment kits, and alternatives to conventional medicine). They are demanding more information on the clinical performance and satisfaction ratings of various health plans and providers before choosing one or the other for their and their families' health care. They are becoming quite militant about managed-care plans perceived to have "gag clauses," "drive-through" deliveries and mastectomies, and gatekeepers (see the earlier discussion). They also are becoming increasingly vocal against for-profit health care organizations of any type that appear to be more interested in shareholders than patients.

Other trends are becoming evident in the purchaser and payer communities. Purchasers are starting to realize that putting the quality of health care first is the best way to ensure both future cost containment and improved patient satisfaction. They are beginning to differentiate competing health plans and provider groups on the basis of their commitment to and successful execution of this "quality-first" philosophy. They are coming to recognize that although health care has its own unique attributes and should not be regarded as a commodity, it nevertheless may be evaluated in much the same way as other major suppliers. These evaluations focus not only on the cost, but, more importantly, on the value of various care options concerning the improvement of the health, productivity, and satisfaction of employees and their families (see Chapter 9).

Finally, there are definite trends among provider groups seeking to reclaim some control over their professional destinies. First, they are consolidating into increasingly larger groups to contend with the ever-larger purchaser groups with which they must bargain. Second, they are assuming the risk of the health and outcomes of the patient populations they serve or are proposing to serve.

The upshot of these trends is that providers must embrace increasingly sophisticated methods for identifying, evaluating, and projecting the needs of populations and subpopulations of patients. Having achieved this, they must identify and implement those evidence-based practices most likely to result in patient outcomes and costs that will not exceed their risk-sharing allowances. They must also be able to document these populations' improvements in clinical outcomes and satisfaction to continue to serve them in the future. Succeeding in all of this is the realm of DM as THM, as developed in this chapter and throughout this book.

Obstacles To Overcome

An entire chapter could be devoted to the obstacles to successful DM implementation. The major obstacles may be grouped into three categories:

1. information technology (IT) and management shortfalls
2. practitioner (especially physician) resistance
3. impatience

The information needs to support DM are discussed in much greater detail in Chapter 4, and especially Chapter 5. Suffice it to say here that the major IT stumbling block is and will continue to be the lack of a standardized computerized patient record in the vast majority of health care organizations. The information from the medical record continues to be the best primary source for evaluating patients' diseases, conditions, severities of illness, diagnostic and therapeutic interventions, results, and progress. Until this information may be recorded, captured, aggregated in a single repository, "sliced and diced," and analyzed in a standardized, systematic manner, DM will provide more potential than actual performance.

The next major obstacle to the success of DM as THM concerns the resistance of physicians and other practitioners. Whether the process is called *disease management, care management, quality management, outcomes management,* or *total health management,* physicians and other practitioners recoil at the notion that anybody or anything might be engaged in *patient* management besides themselves. Consequently, many have regarded DM as merely the latest intrusion into the sacrosanct physician-patient relationship.

Most DM failures can be traced to the lack of input from practitioners into DM design and proposed intervention plans. A reaction to this is for many involved in DM merely to add some "bells and whistles" to previously created patient and physician education programs and to call the result "DM." However, DM as THM necessarily requires much more extensive interventions in the diagnosis, evaluation, and medical management process. Hence, to do DM as THM will require practitioners to be active participants and partners in the DM initiative design and development process.

The final major obstacle to the success of DM as THM is lack of patience among both those involved in doing DM and those intended to benefit from these initiatives. Currently, DM is a source of disillusionment for those practitioners and beneficiaries who had unrealistic expectations concerning the magnitude and speed of its results.

Those who had these unrealistic expectations dashed have either moved on or hunkered down to deal with their "new reality" as best they can. However, those who did recognize from the outset that DM (especially as THM) is a systematic, knowledge-based process that transforms organizations into stakeholder-driven enterprises will continue their commitments and investments that ultimately will be paid back many times.

SUMMARY AND PROSPECTUS

This first chapter was intended to define and begin to develop DM as a knowledge-based, systematic process of evaluating the clinical and related processes. Supported by the best evidence, DM should transform health care delivery into a stakeholder-driven culture capable of producing optimal results for the lowest expenditure of resources. This chapter defined what DM is and is not (or should not be). It outlined why DM is so vital now. It analyzed DM's components, goals, and objectives and evaluated the needs of all of DM's stakeholders: patients, practitioners, providers, product producers, payers, purchasers, and policy makers (the "seven Ps").

DM was discussed not merely as a new methodology but as a new ethic in health care delivery. It was discussed (as it will be in subsequent chapters) as a means for transforming clinical decision making from that most closely associated with the fee-for-service cottage industry of yesterday to that of the (largely) capitated, integrated system of delivery and financing of the near future in this country.

The next four chapters will discuss the various components of DM:

1. its evidence (or knowledge) base
2. practice guidelines (as a means of standardizing practice to those patterns validated as associated with superior outcomes)
3. outcomes measurement and management
4. the information infrastructure

The concluding five chapters will focus on DM as it is actually being applied within or on behalf of the following stakeholders:

1. integrated delivery systems
2. managed-care organizations
3. pharmaceutical firms
4. employers and other major purchasers
5. patients

Finally, in the epilogue to this book, U.S. Senator Bill Frist (the first physician U.S. senator in seven decades, himself a heart and lung transplant surgeon) will discuss the future of DM and the role of policy makers in supporting it. Senator Frist will conclude the book from the perspective of one who has moved along a path similar to that along which DM may be leading the health care industry— from dealing with one patient at a time to determining how best to serve the needs of large populations.

CHAPTER 2

Evidence-Based Medicine

Tony Felton

This chapter is concerned with evidence-based medicine (EBM), its influence on medical practice, and its relationship to disease management.

The perspective of this chapter is to look beyond the "evidence base" itself and to explore how EBM is viewed within the current climate of health reforms, the steps that would be necessary to encourage its wider application, and the strategic implications this is likely to have for health care. We seek to place the development of EBM within the context of the rapid changes in health services seen by doctors and health professionals. Later on in the chapter, we set out to examine attitudes to the evidence itself, its communication, and how EBM may be applied in practice. We then evaluate how EBM is likely to affect the key constituents of health care: payers, providers, patients, and suppliers.

The chapter concludes by analyzing the scope for innovation through the application of disease management driven by EBM. This includes new ways of working through partnerships, information technology, applications of outcomes research, and redesign of the clinical process. We finish by drawing a possible scenario for the future of health care and how this is likely to be shaped by the widespread application of EBM.

DEFINING EBM

Defining EBM presents problems similar to those of defining disease management. Sackett defines EBM as "the contentious, explicit and judicious use of current best evidence in making decisions about the care of individual patients."[1(p 71)] In this definition, *best evidence* is described as "clinically relevant research (especially patient centered clinical research) into the accuracy and precision of diagnostic testing, prognostic markers as well as the efficacy and safety of therapeutic, rehabilitative and preventive regimes."[1(p 71)]

Other definitions of EBM go beyond this, giving a more generalized description that includes "the rigorous evaluation of the effectiveness of healthcare interventions, dissemination of the results of the evaluation and use of the findings to influence clinical practice."[2]

BACKGROUND OF EBM

Medicine predates science, and some aspects of medicine have been important milestones in the development of the scientific method. For example, the processes of hypothesis formation, careful observation, and testing of hypothesis against observation all owe much to the practice of medicine. However, medicine may also be described as an art. Based on an understanding of the whole patient from physical, psychological, and social perspectives, the treatment of disease may be driven as much by experience and intuition as by a purely scientific approach.

By the 19th century, careful observation of patterns of diseases (especially infectious diseases, such as cholera and typhoid, and their association with environmental conditions) led to the emergence of epidemiology and public health medicine. EBM could be said to have been born.

More recently, champions of EBM such as Archie Cochrane sought to establish a more comprehensive scientific approach to medical practice. Thus, the pioneers of EBM set about identifying sources of scientific evidence and used them to influence their colleagues in changing their clinical behavior. However, many factors have impeded the scientific approach to clinical medicine. These include the incomplete nature of the knowledge base and difficulty in gaining access to it as well as the fear that such a "scientific approach" would depersonalize medicine to the detriment of patients and the medical profession.

Nevertheless, as we approach the 21st century, there is a growing body of opinion that medicine practiced according to tradition and judgment alone is inadequate. Because of the rate of scientific advance in so many medical fields, as well as rapid developments in information technology, barriers are falling as to the limitations of the knowledge base itself and its availability. Many doctors welcome a change in their practice and an opportunity to strive for higher standards and improved outcomes for their patients.

We know from our definition of disease management that the key objective of this process is to improve the quality of health outcomes at acceptable cost for specific disease states. Disease management is therefore a broad concept that involves a holistic view of disease from screening and prevention to end stage. It seeks to optimize management at every step.

Applying disease management principles in practice necessitates the use of various supporting processes, including

- *Patient care pathways.* These are used to apply the accepted "best-practice" approach to managing patients with specific conditions (based on the best available evidence and fitting the local environment and culture).
- *Clinical guidelines.* These are systematically developed statements used to assist decision making by health professionals and patients. They may be applied at various stages of a patient care pathway and again are based on the best available evidence. The objective of applying clinical guidelines is to make the appropriate health care interventions for specific clinical circumstances.
- *Clinical protocols.* These are specific and correctly defined processes to be applied in particular clinical circumstances for which little variation or interpretation in practice is necessary (for example, the treatment of ventricular fibrillation).

The application of EBM supports every stage of these processes. It is critical in providing the core knowledge base for an optimal approach to treatment.

If the desire to practice medicine based on scientific evidence is not enough, other forces are pushing the profession in this direction as well. First, the threat of litigation is causing physicians to feel more vulnerable about basing their practice on tradition and judgment not underpinned by scientific evidence. Second, patients themselves, through consumer groups, disease-specific organizations, and the media, are demanding to know more about what treatments are available and the likely risks and outcomes. Finally, with pressure on resources at unprecedented levels, policy makers in some European countries and elsewhere have focused on EBM as one way of prioritizing health care resources.[3] Their belief rests on the notion that by applying rigorous scientific evaluation to current treatments and new treatments, ineffective treatments can be discontinued (Figure 2–1).

In spite of the growing medical knowledge base through such bodies as the UK Cochrane Center, systematic analysis of costs associated with medical interventions is at a very early stage of development. Many commentators believe that such comparative analysis of the costeffectiveness of different interventions is required to support priority setting and resource allocation.[4] There is, however, an assumption among some policy makers that EBM will provide a means to control health care costs.

FROM THEORY TO PRACTICE?

There is little opposition to the theory of EBM. Indeed, it is undeniable that good medical practice should be based whenever possible on scientific evidence. However, if the application of EBM imposes bureaucratic constraints on physi-

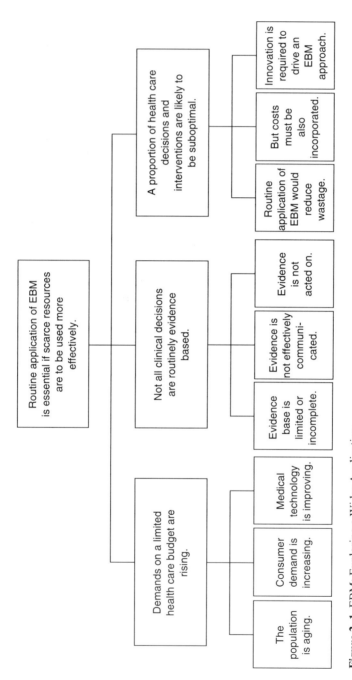

Figure 2–1 EBM: Exploring a Wider Application

cians, many may argue that medicine stands to lose more than it will gain. In particular, if EBM is seen as a way of limiting the costs of health care, it will be rejected by many physicians as not necessarily being in the best interests of patients.

History shows us that the gulf between medical research and clinical practice has often been wide enough to swallow up research that would have provided significant benefit if only it had been put into practice. Reasons for this disconnect are numerous, but two key issues have been identified. First, medical research does not always address issues that are directly relevant to routine medical practice. Second, the results of the research are not always presented in a form that can be readily understood and used.[5]

A number of steps need to be taken to bring EBM into practice (Figure 2–2), especially establishing a validated knowledge base and communicating these findings to change clinical behavior. A continuous improvement feedback loop must link the last and first stages by measuring the actual outcomes of the patient and comparing these with predicted outcomes. Further, changing clinical behavior depends crucially upon the attitude of physicians to the information generated by these steps.

A number of key factors, however, have brought us to the dawn of the age of EBM. Physicians (and patients) themselves are interested in basing their practice on a systematic application of evidence. Moreover, the changing nature of research itself and the growing number of sources of evidence and ease of transmission of this information through computer networks are allowing evidence to be more readily accessed to serve as the foundation for scientifically based medical practice.

New Responsibilities

In recent years, the desire to control rising health care costs in the United States has led to the development of managed care. This continues to affect health systems throughout the world. In this context, EBM provides a very valuable basis for a medical model that can be used to define more precisely the outcomes expected for given inputs. It also provides a basis for discussion between payers and providers, namely, the most appropriate pattern of care and delivery for local needs.

New responsibilities emerging from a managed-care environment have allowed many physicians to step back from individual patient decision making to consider health care from a more strategic perspective and thereby address the needs of patient groups more effectively. EBM is an important tool for this task in that it provides a framework for reevaluating established practices, considering the wider needs of the patient community, and redirecting the work of the clinical team.

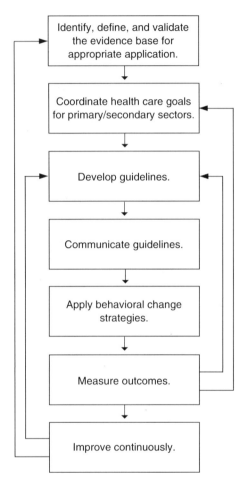

Figure 2–2 Key Steps in the EBM Process. Courtesy of Coopers & Lybrand, London, England.

The recently launched journal *Evidence-Based Medicine* is jointly published by the *British Medical Journal* (*BMJ*) and the American College of Physicians (ACP). Its stated objective is "to bring the best evidence from clinical and healthcare research to the bedside, surgery, clinic and community." The joint nature of the publication is reflected by its editorial board, made up of individuals from North America and the United Kingdom and from a variety of different clinical backgrounds. Much of the content of the journal is taken from the Journal Club of the ACP.

The articles contained in the journal include systematic reviews of health care (often overviews or meta-analyses in which trial results are statistically combined). Clearly, applying the results of an evidence-based review is dependent on the nature and culture of the local health care system. However, it is significant that the international nature of the journal *Evidence-Based Medicine* is likely to raise awareness of best practice on both sides of the Atlantic and to challenge existing paradigms concerning the purchasing and provision of health care.

In the United States, health-related information is widely available to the public. With rising expectations for health care outcomes, a failure to deliver best practice will increasingly be challenged by individual patients and patient groups. Those who are involved in managing care programs are aware of patients' interest in achieving and improving outcomes. Shortcomings due to cost reduction or substandard practice are unlikely to be tolerated by consumers.

EBM in the United States therefore is becoming a yardstick for health care. With the advancement of information technology, information related to best-practice health care is rapidly becoming accessible not only to health professionals but to the population at large.

Management Control and the Threat of Litigation

One effect of the health care reforms has been the loss of the autonomy that many physicians have enjoyed for so long. The introduction of managed care means that health care decisions can no longer be seen as simply the aggregation of many individual professional choices. Health care will henceforth be defined in relation to needs, described in contracts, and managed to fulfill those contracts. For the physician, this means that some sort of management control will replace personal autonomy in many spheres.

As a result, many physicians have a sense of being controlled by a management that is often remote from and insensitive to the pressures of working in a demanding clinical setting. Alongside this is a feeling of loss of the job security and lifetime employment that medicine traditionally provided.

At the same time, the threat of litigation is increasing as both the incidence of claims and the costs of meeting claims rise rapidly (as has been demonstrated by the rapid rise in medical insurance costs in recent years). In this context, following EBM guidelines may provide some shelter to clinical teams. If, however, EBM becomes a defensive barrier to litigation, significant costs could be incurred to safeguard against *all* possible events as opposed to likely eventualities. EBM also raises questions regarding legal responsibilities. If a claim arises for a case in which an agreed-on guideline has been followed, it is not always clear how responsibility should be apportioned between those who developed and approved the guideline and those who followed it.[6]

Changing Patterns of Care

In many countries, major health care reforms of the last 5 years have resulted in a steady shift of patient care from traditional hospital-based services to community and general-practice care. This has partly been driven by medical advances that have cut the length of hospital stay or enabled patients to be maintained and monitored in the community rather than in the hospital. Such trends are particularly evident in the management of mental illness and chronic diseases such as asthma, diabetes, and some forms of cancer.

EBM provides a framework for systematically reviewing and defining current knowledge of best practice in all sectors of health care. As such, there is a danger that it can be misused simply as a recipe for transferring responsibilities. Properly applied, it can support joint planning and provision of care. Since EBM encourages a detailed focus on the patient at each stage in treatment and care, it should lend itself to integrated care and resource planning. It is here that EBM plays a critical role in the disease management process.

Coping with Time and Resource Constraints

Pressures arising from limited resources are a factor that physicians have had to cope with for many years. With the growing importance of the "gatekeeping" role of the general practitioner, it is likely that such pressures will increase and that conflicts over resources will become more contentious and public. Many physicians are now seeking a more systematic use of objective evidence to guide them on how to apply scarce resources most effectively.

Increasing constraints on resources have resulted in less time available for physicians to keep up with medical developments. Medical consultants in the United Kingdom report that they have less than 1 hour a week available for reading medical literature, and many physicians complain they are "drowning" in a rising tide of medical literature.[7] EBM may assist physicians in this task by providing access to such knowledge and enabling them to find out what is best practice. For some patients, the prospect of a physician's turning to a book or computer for guidance is reassuring. For others, it may undermine confidence. These issues need to be examined carefully if the benefits of EBM are to be accepted by physicians and their patients.

How Patients' Demands Are Changing

Patient demands are growing for three main reasons. First, the proportion of very elderly patients (age 75 and older) continues to rise. The demands on physicians resulting from the growth of the elderly population has become a significant issue throughout the developed world. This is compounded by limitations in availability of residential care, the breakup of the nuclear family, and less willingness to look after elderly relatives.

Second, the development of medical technology—from surgical intervention to advanced diagnostic and therapeutic agents—has encouraged patients to seek medical treatment that would not have been available in the past.

Third, patients are acting more like consumers, with rising expectations of quality, levels of service, and information. Coverage of medical issues by the media has helped to raise levels of awareness among the population and to increase ease of access to medical information and higher levels of education. Some patients believe that physicians' decisions are driven by external factors such as budgets and formularies rather than what is in the patients' best interests. In certain countries, this has led to a growing distrust of physicians and a weakening of the traditional physician-patient relationship.

EBM can be seen as a basis for explaining physicians' decisions to patients. However, such use of EBM requires not only that guidelines be explained in a relevant way to patients but also that an EBM process provide a better way of listening to patients, understanding their needs, and empowering them with objective evidence to contribute to decisions that may be taken on their behalf.

EBM guidelines should be concerned with the care provided by patients themselves and their nonprofessional caregivers as part of overall management. The evidence on which EBM is based must therefore reflect the patients' perspective. Outcomes cannot simply be evaluated in medical terms but must also consider the physical, psychological, and social perspectives of patients themselves.

PHYSICIANS AND EBM

In the United States, disease management is currently having a significant impact on the provision of health care. This is likely to grow in coming years and spread to other countries. However, the concept of disease management has met with some resistance from the medical profession, particularly in Europe. The threats of management control, commercialization of health care, and loss of patient confidentiality have generated suspicion and hostility.

The concept of EBM, although a key component of disease management, appears to be more palatable to many physicians. A crucial benefit that is likely to arise from both disease management and EBM is greater collaboration between different parties concerned with improving quality and effectiveness of health care delivery across traditionally held boundaries.

The history of EBM led us to believe that the attitudes of physicians would be crucial not only to the general acceptance of the concept but also to its application in practice.[8] We therefore set out to answer four simple questions:

1. What evidence do physicians see as relevant?
2. Is the evidence effectively communicated?
3. Is the evidence acted on?
4. Are physicians' attitudes to EBM favorable or unfavorable?

Behind these primary questions lies the desire to explore what research key individuals are implementing, what "levers" may be used to influence change, and what examples of EBM best practice currently exist. To answer these questions, we conducted a survey of 506 physicians in the United Kingdom who represented both general-practice and hospital medicine.[8]

What Evidence Do Physicians See as Relevant?

The first part of our definition of EBM is "the rigorous evaluation of the effectiveness of health care interventions." The evidence required for such evaluation is itself diverse and may arise from a variety of sources. It includes evidence of the resources required to carry out a medical intervention. It can simplistically be split into four domains: evidence gained from (1) controlled clinical trials, (2) medical observational data, (3) patient observational data, and (4) cost data (Figure 2–3).

Randomized controlled clinical trials are generally perceived as the the the "gold standard" of the evidence base. Even within that body of evidence, however, questions relating to the validity of particular trials, trial results, and relevance of results to local populations need to be carefully assessed before the evidence can be properly applied. At the other end of the continuum, individual case histories are generally perceived as the weakest source of evidence. But when health professionals are asked directly what constitutes a relevant knowledge base for them, they respond with a far broader definition of the evidence base than might be expected. From our survey, we found the following:[8]

- Clinical outcome evidence, followed by controlled trial data, was the most powerful influence for general practitioners (GPs) in persuading them to change clinical practice.
- Data recorded by patients themselves are likely to become a more important influence on physician practice.
- Only one third of our respondents spent more than 1 hour a week reading medical literature.

For a more detailed discussion of these issues, please refer to Chapter 3.

Is the Evidence Effectively Communicated?

From our survey, we found the following:[8]

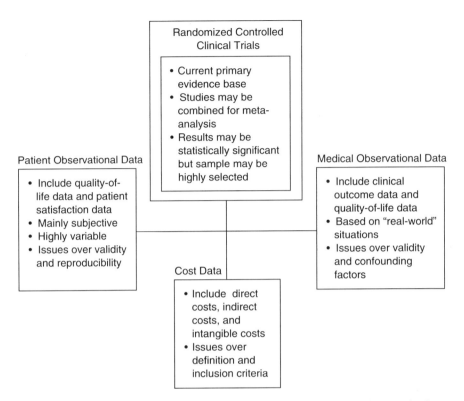

Figure 2–3 Domains of Evidence. Courtesy of Coopers & Lybrand, London, England.

- Most hospital physicians were using or were intending to use the EBM process for review and communication of best practice through development of guidelines and their dissemination.
- EBM was more likely to influence physicians in changing their prescribing behavior than other drug education efforts.
- Nearly three quarters of GP respondents were using or were intending to use EBM to review their clinical practice, and half were conducting or were intending to conduct their own outcome studies.
- Key success factors common to best-practice examples of applying EBM included: well-funded and coordinated projects, involvement of local practitioners, multidisciplinary consensus in guideline development, adequate training, use of incentives, and audit of results.

Many respondents mentioned that they were at a preliminary stage of installing the computer technology required for these tasks. Others were hampered by lack of funds, facilities, or user-friendly systems. CD-ROM and the Internet were identified by a number of respondents as specific technology that will be of growing importance in this area.

Is the Evidence Routinely Applied in Medical Practice?

From the responses, it appears that GPs base their prescribing, treatment, and diagnostics primarily on evidence but that a significant proportion of respondents rarely or never rely on *research* evidence to conduct these activities. Presumably, they use tradition, judgment, and personal experience instead. Further, a significant proportion of respondents do not use research evidence to guide them in purchasing or making referrals.

From our survey, we found the following:[8]

- Most respondents believed that improving patient outcomes was the best reason to apply EBM.
- Most respondents agreed that EBM was likely to improve clinical practice but that a reduction in flexibility was likely.
- Barriers to applying EBM included lack of time, expertise, access to evidence, and validation of outcome evidence.

Overall Attitudes to EBM

In response to a question about what would influence physicians to embrace an EBM, improvement of patient outcomes was, not surprisingly cited as the most powerful "lever," followed by the possibility of better access to EBM summaries. Our hypothesis from the outset of the study was that the attitude of physicians to EBM was of critical importance to the subsequent adoption and application of EBM initiatives. Responses from our survey seemed to signal a high degree of enthusiasm toward EBM and a belief that its application was likely to bring about enhanced patient care and job satisfaction. Nevertheless, a small but significant proportion of respondents remained unconvinced of its merits.

Some respondents highlighted the possible misuse of EBM, particularly by parties outside medicine, trying to justify policy changes. Many comments were made regarding difficulty in accessing evidence at the time it was needed. This was particularly true in primary care and ranked as a key barrier for limiting the adoption of EBM.

A number of respondents pointed out that patients do not present in neat, uniform ways and that EBM was only one element in the treatment of the whole patient's needs. A common cry was one of limited time available to get started in applying EBM, even at the most basic level. This sentiment was echoed by a plea for help from outside sources such as public health consultants and hospital consultants with specific interests in this area.

Further warnings came from a number of respondents over the "regimentation" of the approach to medicine that EBM might bring, thereby limiting medical advancement. Many respondents also commented on the nature and selection of the evidence, stating that it was essential to establish its validity and clear definition before interpretation.

In summary, we believe that as the awareness of EBM spreads to the majority of physicians, a more positive attitude is likely to develop, from which a more active involvement in EBM activities may arise.

HOW WILL EBM AFFECT KEY CONSTITUENTS WITHIN HEALTH CARE?

It is at present unclear whether EBM will be routinely adopted as standard practice in all parts of medicine. Even if its adoption across the medical spectrum is limited, it is already having an impact on key constituents of the health services. This trend is likely to increase and extend to groups outside the immediate domain of health care purchasing and provision to include patients themselves and suppliers, particularly the pharmaceutical industry (Figure 2–4).

Payers and Purchasers

As payers attempt to purchase clinically effective interventions and reduce ineffective ones,[9] they need to bring together the diverse services provided by acute, community, and primary care providers into an integrated package of patient-focused care. Payers not only must attempt to define such packages but also must act as change agents working with health care providers to introduce new patterns of services provision.[10]

An example of how EBM has been applied in practice is the GRIPP (Getting Research into Practice and Purchasing) project. Centered in the Oxford region of the United Kingdom, GRIPP set out to incorporate research into practice through the purchasing process and by raising patient awareness. One example was the objective of reducing the level of D&C operations (dilatation and curettage of the uterus) in women under age 40 (a common procedure that had been shown to confer limited medical benefit). After evidence-based guidelines had been developed by a multidisciplinary group, information was given to the public and GPs to outline the risks and limited benefits of the treatment. By these means, and by the coordinated efforts of local purchasers, local GPs, and acute care providers, a 57% reduction in D&C rates was achieved.[11]

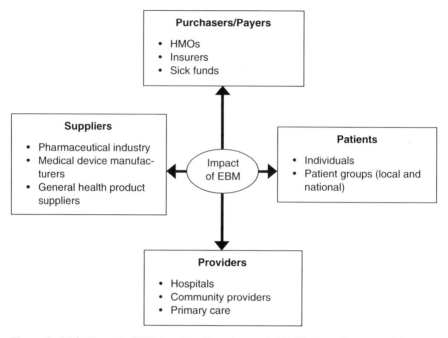

Figure 2–4 The Impact of EBM on Key Constituents in Health Care. Courtesy of Coopers & Lybrand, London, England.

Central to the notion of evidence-based purchasing is measurement of inputs and outcomes. Indeed, many commentators believe that the whole health care quality movement is likely to be absorbed in a wider quality initiative that will encompass EBM. This can already be observed in the United States, where the development of managed care has given rise to the concept of "value purchasing."[12] This concept has been used strategically to raise quality standards through the following methodologies:

- a predefined specification and measurement of quality and cost-effectiveness between purchasers and providers
- comparable and agreed-upon severity-adjusted standards
- agreed-upon selection criteria of providers based on clinical performance
- incentives to direct contracting and to reward high-value providers

Such a rational approach is likely to require considerably better information systems than are currently available in most European health care systems. The recurring theme, however, even in the competitive environment in which medicine is practiced in the United States, is that partnership and longer-term cooperation between purchasers and providers are the best approach to improving communication, information flow, and, ultimately, quality standards.

Health Care Providers

Communication of evidence such as systematic reviews, meta-analysis, and examples of best practice remained a barrier for many respondents of our survey. For many, the necessary information technology was either not available or in early stages of evolution. Paper-based systems remained the most common form of information interchange. The medical literature was still the most important means of communicating this kind of information.

Given the importance of direct contact between clinical colleagues as an important source of evidence, appropriate networks need to be developed and extended to further this contact at a local level, especially to bridge the secondary-primary care divide. In practice, this may mean supporting facilities to enable hospital physicians, GPs, and other professional staff, possibly through joint training initiatives, to form stronger local networks. Indeed, some medical educators would go further by recommending that the undergraduate and postgraduate medical curriculum should include the learning of techniques to access and assimilate information necessary to develop an evidence-based approach to medical practice.

Benchmarking health provider organizations is likely to highlight areas where evidence-based practice is currently lacking and those that demonstrate particular examples of good practice. A simple framework for benchmarking services can identify

- services that are already meeting needs most effectively
- services that should be moving toward prevention to improve cost-effectiveness
- services whose cost-effectiveness could be improved by better coordination among providers
- services whose cost-effectiveness could be improved by altering the type of service provided

With this simple framework, EBM initiatives may be prioritized in a systematic way, and progress may be benchmarked with other organizations.

So far, we have largely concentrated upon physicians, but we must also acknowledge the important role that nurses have to play in EBM. Nurses not only carry out many of the tasks dictated by EBM protocols but also bring a very important dimension to EBM based on their skills and experience in caregiving. A recent study of nurse practitioners concludes that a multidisciplinary approach to the delivery of services improves patient outcomes and can be enhanced by nursing approaches to care.[13] These include the ability to develop long-term relationships with patients and to support self-care and family care. Nurse practitioners can also provide aspects of medical care within safe boundaries defined by evidence-based protocols (including prescribing and compliance programs).

Ward-based, primary care, and community-based nurses can support each other in ensuring continuity of care within an EBM environment. Indeed, our own experiences suggest that nurses can exchange information on the expected progress of a patient's care and his or her actual outcome with fewer barriers to communication than in physician-to-physician exchanges. In most cases, the eventual outcome for patients is a resumption of daily living with greater or lesser impairment to function. Nurses are often more able to capture such information.

Patients

Attitudes and expectations among patients have changed in recent years. No longer are most members of the public satisfied to "get what they are given" if this is deemed to fall below their expectations. Increasingly, calls are made in the media to improve public understanding and allow patients to have greater involvement in issues of choice by explaining the basis for medical decisions.[14]

One of the challenges facing payers is to create better understanding between the public and health service providers. This must be the basis for determining health care priorities and for involving the public both in their own self-care and in the choice of treatment modes. The public also need to be given clear expectations of the standard and quality of services they should expect so that they may become the most important levers for service improvement.

Patient interest groups are now well informed and vocal, demanding to have greater involvement in issues such as research directions, incorporation of treatment into practice, and improvement in patients' quality of life. Dangers exist if the provision of services is based on the lobbying abilities of specific patient groups. We would argue that this risk points to an even greater need for making decisions based on evidence.

The role of employers in influencing local health care provision is of less importance in Europe than in North America. Nevertheless, because the cost of absenteeism in some industries is a burden that employers wish to address in a more active way, EBM is likely to be used in the context of reviewing employees' health, especially in assessing the value of screening and prevention services. Private health insurance is one benefit that many employers provide for their work force. Private providers are pioneering the use of EBM methods to evaluate the cost-effectiveness of interventions that they deliver or finance.

The development of patient information presents two challenges: the collection of information from patients themselves on their experience and outcomes and the dissemination of evidence-based information to patients for the purpose of involving them in their treatment and care decisions. From our survey, it appears that physicians are indeed basing some of their decisions on evidence of patient outcomes. As "efficacy" gives way to "effectiveness," patient-focused outcome data assume strategic importance. Clearly, issues such as defining patient outcomes and end points need to be standardized before such research can have widespread applicability. However, agreement on these issues will in itself help to highlight what outcomes are important from the patient's perspective. This should focus needs accordingly.

In Europe, collection of outcomes data remains hampered by uncertainties in the law regarding confidentiality. However, the creation of large patient databases, such as the IMS Mediplus database, based on GP and hospital treatment and outcome data, is already providing a source of valuable information. In the future, this will support evidence from more traditional areas in the formulation of best-practice guidelines.

Providing information for patients (such as written instructions for patients after a head injury) has gone on for many years. The advancement of technology has enabled such information to be made available in a more user-friendly way (such as videos on treatments for patients). It is likely that technology will go further, for example, allowing patients to "experience" a treatment through virtual reality systems before agreeing to have it.[15]

In spite of these ideas, many patients rely on physicians' judgments without having the information available to challenge those decisions. As systems such as the Internet extend their coverage, the repository of medical information, traditionally available to the medical profession alone, is opening up to a wider audience. Since this trend is unstoppable, it would appear advisable for the medical profession to seek ways in which they can harness it for improving patient care.

Bringing EBM to the people may be resisted by some within the medical profession who see it as, at best, premature and, at worst, inflating patient expectations to levels that cannot be met. Some may also view EBM as providing a stick to beat physicians with—a development that would be unlikely to improve patient care, given current resource constraints. Yet some forward-looking innovators within the medical profession who see themselves working in a competitive environment are themselves developing this idea as a way of providing a superior service for patients, thereby attracting larger numbers.

Suppliers: The Pharmaceutical and Medical Supply Industries

Disease management is a broad concept that incorporates EBM while (1) encouraging prevention, (2) maximizing clinical effectiveness, (3) eliminating ineffective or unnecessary care, (4) using only cost-effective diagnosis and therapeutics, (5) maximizing the efficiency of care delivery, and (6) encouraging continuous improvement. Figure 2–5 shows the spectrum of care over which the disease management process can be applied.

Why has the pharmaceutical industry become so interested in disease management? Disease management challenges the stable business environment and presents both a threat and an opportunity. The threat arises from the fear that products supplied by some companies may not be found to be cost-effective once a thorough EBM evaluation has taken place.[16] Lack of cost-effectiveness would mean that even if a product met necessary safety and efficacy specifications, its market would be likely to diminish. Some countries such as Australia and Canada have gone further and regulated the price by which new drugs may gain reimbursement, based on the new product's cost-effectiveness compared to that of existing comparable agents. As the reality of price controls and diminishing markets haunts some companies, others see the opportunity to move out of their traditional product-oriented business and to provide a far broader portfolio of products and services based on addressing the needs of customers in a particular therapeutic area in which that company may have core expertise. The best examples of disease management so far have involved chronic diseases such as asthma, diabetes, and cancer. Some innovative companies are now considering applying disease management principles to broader therapeutic categories such as infection control and fertility management.

From the supplier's perspective, there are three keys to applying EBM principles to further disease management: first, gaining access to outcome data on which to base these services; second, developing interventions such as guidelines and educational materials with which to implement such a program; and third, forming partnerships with providers and other parties to execute such a program.

Lower Costs ◄	Spectrum of Care		► Higher Costs

Disease Management

Self-Directed	Primary	Secondary	Tertiary	Long-Term
Patients Prevention Home care	Primary care Physicians/ allied health professionals	Specialist Outpatient clinics	Hospitals/ centers of excellence	Institutions Nursing homes

Figure 2–5 Spectrum of Care for Applications of the Disease Management Process. Courtesy of Coopers & Lybrand, London, England.

In this way, a more systematic assessment of unmet needs may be made that is likely to enhance market value and product positioning and to provide a means of improving value to health service customers and patients.

Some pharmaceutical companies are therefore shifting their strategic focus from product research, development, and marketing to provision of health care services in specific therapeutic areas. This radical shift is likely to alter profoundly the internal and external role of companies that choose it. Internally, not only does it require new skills, (i.e., information systems and services), but it is likely to alter fundamental processes such as product research, development, and marketing. For instance, the sales representative force is more likely to be involved with working with providers to set up information systems, implement guidelines, and run educational programs than to promote products by direct sales to users.

Externally, the industry will need to form longer-term partnerships with its customers. Pharmaceutical companies have a rich repository of skills and resources at their disposal with which they can assist customers in furthering their efforts toward EBM. These include pharmacoeconomic expertise, data management skills, communication and education experience, a sales force, finance, a global presence, research methodology experience, and, perhaps, a willingness to take risks. Leading companies will use these resources to find ways of addressing their customers' needs, thereby building closer relationships.

A further trend that is beginning to emerge in the United States may involve the sharing of risk between companies and their customers. Although this idea has been discussed for some time, the data necessary for such risk-sharing agreements are still at a preliminary stage of development. However, one can envision a time in which a company wishing to launch a new and expensive product might be required to accept some financial risk on behalf of a customer if the product failed to meet given specifications. Clearly, the existence of a comprehensive disease management program based on evidence is essential if costs are to be controlled and if the effectiveness of the new agent is to be optimized. Nevertheless, such initiatives are likely to be short lived if physicians are not convinced of their value for themselves and their patients.

The idea of the health care value chain can help to explain how the role and function of the pharmaceutical industry are likely to alter. The value chain is a simple method of disaggregating steps in a process or service that add to the value of that service for a customer or user. Figure 2–6 shows a "traditional" health value chain, with the pharmaceutical company at the top, followed by its prime customer (the provider), followed by the purchaser, and finally the patient. Key to this process is the discovery, manufacture, and sale of products that generate revenue necessary to keep this system going.

Figure 2–7 shows a "new" health value chain that has been turned upside down and back to front. Here, the patient is at the top of the chain, and patient

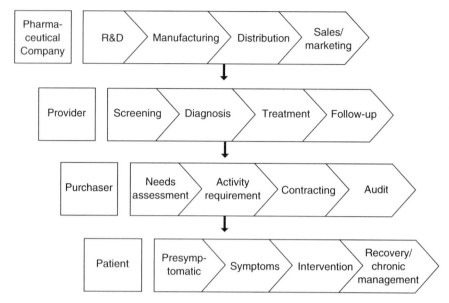

Figure 2–6 Traditional Health Value Chain. Courtesy of Coopers & Lybrand, London, England.

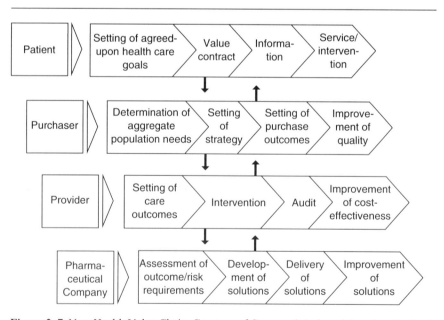

Figure 2–7 New Health Value Chain. Courtesy of Coopers & Lybrand, London, England.

values drive the activity of suppliers. Addressing patient needs while controlling costs is the goal that purchasers, providers, and ultimately the pharmaceutical industry seek to achieve. The value contract acts as the starting point for addressing patient needs, followed up by providers' agreement to deliver agreed-upon outcomes that have been set by purchasers. The role of the pharmaceutical industry therefore shifts to the assessment of outcomes and risk requirements of its provider customers, followed by the development, delivery, and continuous improvement of solutions (which are likely to include products supported by services).

Clearly, major hurdles such as developing long-term partnerships and accessing credible clinical and cost data will have to be overcome if pharmaceutical companies are to become fully involved in disease management and EBM initiatives. Yet within the current climate of change, opportunities for more collaborative work are appearing as fast as old barriers fall.

Irrespective of the impact of disease management on pharmaceutical companies, launching new products in an environment that is increasingly based on evidence is already having a significant effect. This ranges from incorporating EBM into R&D decision making and portfolio management to demonstrating effectiveness in a clinical setting and determining the criteria applied by key decision makers in new product decisions. As payers demand more information from suppliers about their products' effectiveness based on outcome evidence, competitive advantage within the whole industry may rest on companies' ability to transform themselves into fully integrated providers that are focused on addressing patients' needs in the most cost-effective way.[17]

In summary, providing cost-effective solutions is likely to be more efficiently rewarded in the future than it has been in the past. Innovation toward this end is likely to go beyond traditional R&D. It will encompass services, partnerships, and information needs that are customer focused. Pharmaceutical companies will need to base strategies on these tenets if they hope to maintain their competitive advantage.

THE ROLE OF INFORMATION TECHNOLOGY

The importance of information and information technology (IT) in extending EBM cannot be overstated. It links the disparate parts of the network by linking evidence sources to provide end users with information and tools necessary to implement EBM initiatives (Figure 2–8).

Findings from our survey showed that computers are already being used to varying degrees to collate patient data, access guidelines and evidence-based reviews, and exchange knowledge with colleagues. However, in spite of considerable quantities of audit data in secondary and primary care, much of this stays

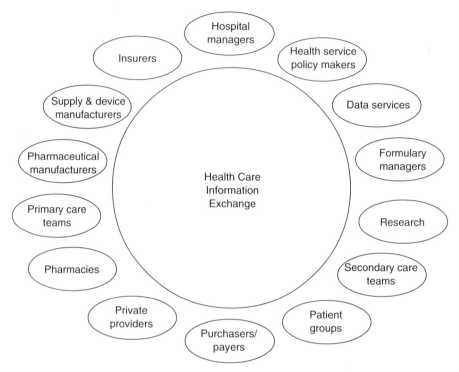

Figure 2–8 Health Care Information Partnerships. Courtesy of Coopers & Lybrand, London, England.

internal, and benefits rarely reach those who collect and enter the data. This situation is likely to improve through a variety of developments. The development of local health care networks (such as the community health information networks in the United States) will considerably facilitate information interchange between constituents at local and national levels (but see Chapter 5 for more recent developments).

The use of IT systems to measure outcomes is likely to increase as part of the continuous improvement of the EBM process. However, issues such as case mix, disease severity indexing, definition of outcome end points, and epidemiological data must be clarified if outcome data studies are to be validated. There have, however, been considerable successes in this field, especially in the development of disease registers such as the UK Heart Valve Registry.[18]

Key success factors in these examples include motivation from clinicians who see clear benefit in the form of research material and improved patient management from the collection of such data. In addition, these successful disease registers usually had a "champion" to coordinate the enterprise and, for the most part, employed user-friendly software to facilitate data exchange.

The Internet is already open to technically minded patients, and it is likely to be increasingly accessed by medical and nonmedical users who seek information such as best-practice guidelines and protocols.[19] Clearly, most users of the Internet, as younger people, are themselves unlikely to require health care services at present. However, in the United States, certain patient groups (particularly HIV/AIDS sufferers) have used this medium very effectively to form self-help networks to exchange information regarding research and best practice. In addition, many people use the Internet as a source of information on behalf of elderly relatives who may be less computer literate. In time, as network technology becomes more accessible to the public at large, direct access to EBM data is likely to become more widespread.

Computers and networks, however, have their limitations when it comes to maintaining patient confidentiality. At present, significant concerns exist in some countries about how such systems may be made secure.[20] But the future points to IT systems that will enable clinicians to access large databases during the consultation and will allow direct comparison of a patient's condition to very large numbers of similar cases. From this comparison, probability of risk from different treatment options may be assessed and agreement reached with the patient on his or her choice of treatment in a way that could not have been achieved in the past.

CREATING AN ENVIRONMENT TO ENCOURAGE EBM

Health reforms have made many physicians wary of management. Concerns have already been voiced about how EBM is another management tool rather than a process for improving patient care. A modern teaching hospital is one of the most complex organizations. It may include more than 100 different professions with advanced knowledge and skills and complex information technology and medical equipment. The needs of each patient are different, and the outcomes of health processes may ultimately be life or death.

In the face of such complexity and uncertainty, management is extremely difficult, if not impossible. Henry Mintzberg,[21] a professor of organizational behavior, proposed a model of hospital organization that recognizes that most of the information required to manage a hospital cannot be captured in "top-down" management instructions. Control is, of necessity, "trained into" the professional health care team.

If EBM is seen as a way of codifying medical practice to the point that it can be readily be subjected to bureaucratic supervision and control, it will inevitably result in defensive behavior and will fail. EBM must be implemented in an organizational context that supports clinical teamwork and encourages communication and learning within and among teams. The relevant organizational model is not one of "command and control" but one of teams empowered by access to knowledge and information and working in a supportive network. This is a model to which many modern organizations now aspire.[22]

An examination of patient care processes can be particularly powerful. It provides an opportunity for primary and secondary clinical teams to reframe their services from the patient's perspective. Often such exercises can immediately identify opportunities to eliminate duplication and delay and to improve patients' experiences. With the added potential of IT for sharing and using medical knowledge and patient information, exceptional improvements can be made.

This approach has five main advantages:

1. It focuses on the central concern of clinical teams for their patients.
2. It creates linkages between the work of different professionals within clinical teams.
3. It does not impose a hierarchical structure but reinforces a working network.
4. It can establish a method for continuously capturing the patients' responses and outcomes and thus can lead to continuous improvement.
5. It develops a creative process that supports clinical teams in solving their own problems rather than imposing cuts and constraints.

This is not meant to imply that there is not a role for management in health care. Both general managers and medical directors have very valuable roles, but they should direct, enable, and support clinical teamwork rather than attempting to impose supervision and control.

NEW WAYS OF WORKING AS A CONSEQUENCE OF EBM

Health care is being shaped by forces external to the medical profession that include technological and economic changes as well as new market demands. These forces are likely to influence the role of the health care professional as well as the health care process itself, particularly in the form of changing interprofessional roles and communication.

The key to the success in developing partnerships that enables EBM to progress is their objective to make life easier, not harder, for those involved. In addition, ensuring flexibility and tailoring EBM programs to the specific needs of subgroups involved must be fundamental objectives. The complexity and diversity of clinical practice will mean that the spread of EBM is likely to be slower than many protagonists hope. However, the payback may be achieved through a more systematic and thorough penetration of the concept. Overall success rests on EBM programs based on a deep understanding of the culture and environment in which evidence-based clinical practice will occur.

New participants such as the pharmaceutical industry, private health care providers, insurance companies, and information companies will enter the picture along with traditional agencies. Their entry will be driven by the increasing sophistication of purchasers and their ability to measure value in terms of inputs, costs, and outcomes. EBM therefore represents a methodology that brings together medical evidence and best practice within a new framework of partnerships between health care professionals and different agencies with the common objective of addressing patients' needs in the most cost-effective way.

LOOKING TO THE FUTURE

In spite of resistance to further change from many in the medical profession, the delivery of health care within the next 5 years is likely to be substantially different from what exists at present. Within primary care, physicians are likely to work in larger networks while developing subspecialist interests that may involve clinical or management functions. Within some health services, physicians will increasingly take on a role as managers of resources that are available for patients. To undertake this task effectively, they will lead increasingly large and diverse health care teams, who will carry out many tasks and activities that are currently undertaken by physicians themselves, such as screening for disease and monitoring of patients with chronic diseases. The evolving role of nurses will be particularly prominent in this domain.

In terms of health care delivery, clinical decision making is likely to be supported by locally agreed-upon guidelines and defined treatment paths for most chronic diseases. Physicians will also have access to large outcome databases that individual patients' conditions will be matched against, and decisions may be made in terms of risks and benefits from the likely outcomes of different management options.

Patients are likely to be more demanding in this decision process and will be directly involved in selecting the option of choice together with their physician or member of the health care team. The role of nurse practitioners is likely to increase substantially. However, patients' involvement in any treatment plan will be more precisely defined, as will be the "minimum standards" of the medical care they can expect. Patients' copayments may be linked to adherence to prescribed guidelines.

Within hospital care, a different pattern of care provision is likely to emerge. As more and more patient management is shifted from hospital to community care, the role of the traditional "general hospital" is likely to diminish. Commensurate with that will be the rise of certain tertiary or super-regional specialist centers, where expertise and technology are likely to be concentrated with the objective of delivering high-quality, cost-effective outcomes with fully integrated services dedicated to the treatment of a particular condition. An example of this may include the management of breast cancer.

Traditional providers will work under tighter cost and outcome controls, as has developed in the U.S. managed-care market. Improvements in IT will enable most local provider units to work in closer collaboration with their purchasers. Provider organizations, and individual clinicians who work within them, are likely to be scrutinized to a far higher degree in terms of their clinical performance as measured by outcomes. Their rewards will in part be linked to outcome measures and will include skill developments arising from the completion of evidence-based continuing medical education programs. The wide variation in outcomes of treatment of patients adjusted for case mix and severity will also come under scrutiny. Less effective treatments will be discarded. The costs of treatment and the cost benefit of outcomes will be routinely monitored and incorporated as part of guidelines and treatment pathways.

Many of these prognostications are likely to raise issues and reactions from the medical profession. However, if physicians fail to rise to the challenge and fulfill a leadership role in an increasingly cost-conscious and standards-driven environment, they will risk becoming marginalized in this debate.

We face an era of expensive new medical technology arising from biotechnology, gene therapy, and advanced diagnostics, as well as rising demands for more traditional treatments. Limitations on resources will challenge all physicians' ability to deliver effective health care that is fair and open to all groups in society. This decision making must rest on scientific evidence, since the complexity of this process extends beyond what individual practitioners can manage through personal judgment and experience. However, the process must also be tailored to the needs of the local environment. It is within this context that EBM is likely to be applied systematically to the purchase and delivery of health care. In the long term, it is likely to enhance benefits to patients that could ultimately be of as much importance as, or even greater importance than, other well-publicized breakthroughs in medical science.

References

1. Sackett D, Rosenberg W, Muir Grey J, Haynes R, Scott Richardson W. Evidence based medicine: what it is and what it isn't. *Br Med J.* 1996;312:71–72.
2. Appleby J, Walshe K, Ham C. *Acting on the Evidence.* NAHAT Research Paper No. 17.
3. UK Labour Party. *Renewing the NHS: Labour's Agenda for a Healthier Britain.*
4. 80% of NHS treatments simply may not work. *Mail on Sunday.* June 15, 1995.

5. Owens P. Clinical practice and medical research: bridging the divide between two cultures. *Br J Gen Prac*. October 1995;45:557–560.

6. Hurwitz B. Clinical guidelines and the law. *Br Med J*. 1995;311:1517–1518.

7. Sackett DL. Surveys of self-reported reading times of consultants in Oxford, Birmingham, Milton Keynes, Bristol, Leicester and Glasgow. In: Sackett DL, Richardson WS, Rosenberg WMC, Haynes RB, eds. *Evidence Based Medicine: How to Practice and Teach EBM*. London: Churchill Livingstone; 1997.

8. Felton T, Lister G. *Consider the Evidence*. London: Coopers and Lybrand; 1996.

9. Hayward J. Purchasing clinically effective care. *Br Med J*. 1994;309:823–824.

10. Owen N. *Re-engineering the Purchasing Strategy*. Healthfile No 4, December 1995.

11. Getting Research into Practice and Purchasing. *Getting Research into Practice and Purchasing: Resource Pack*. Anglia and Oxford Regional Health Authority; 1994.

12. Couch JB. Health care quality management for the 21st century. *Am Coll Physician Executives*. 1991;129.

13. Tofts A. *Partnerships for Change: Working To Develop Primary Care*. 1995.

14. Maxwell RJ. A careful prescription. *Financial Times*. October 30, 1995.

15. Meredith P, Emberton M, Wood C. New directions in information for patients *Br Med J*. 1995;311:4–5.

16. Warner P, Cooper M. Taking stock. *Health Serv*. October 26, 1995:33.

17. Freemantle N, Henry D, Maynard A, Torrance G. Promoting cost effective prescribing. *Br Med J*. 1995;310:955–956.

18. Taylor K. Take heart. *Br J Healthcare Comput*. May 1991.

19. Coiera E. The Internet's challenge to healthcare provision. *Br Med J*. 1996;3:2–3.

20. Anderson R. NHS-wide networking and patient confidentiality. *Br Med J*. 1995;311:5–6.

21. Mintzberg H. *Structure in Fives*. New York, NY: Prentice Hall; 1988.

22. Moss Kanter R. *When Giants Learn To Dance*. New York, NY: Simon & Schuster; 1989.

CHAPTER 3

Outcome-Validated Clinical Practice Guidelines: A Scientific Foundation for Disease Management

Scott Weingarten and Geneen Graber

Clinical practice guidelines are being used widely in health care today. There currently exist multiple constituencies that are developing and implementing practice guidelines on national, state, and local levels. With the latest American Medical Association report revealing that over 2000 guidelines have already been developed by approximately 75 organizations,[1] it is clear that the guideline movement is flourishing. As clinicians, we must understand why and how guidelines are developed. But even more important, we need to establish that each guideline can assist clinicians in improving patient care and achieving optimal efficiency. We must prove that guidelines represent the best possible care for patients. Clinicians are most likely to accept guidelines if these are tested and proved both safe and effective through measurement of patient outcomes.

Disease management programs may include guidelines. With the recent economic and structural changes in the health care system, disease management may become a fundamental component of patient care. The eventual success or failure of the disease management program may depend, in part, on the effectiveness of guidelines when translated into clinical practice.

This chapter will address the following issues:

- issues related to inappropriate health care
- past attempts to redress the inappropriate utilization of resources
- the concept of disease management and physicians' attitudes toward it
- the concept of clinical practice guidelines and their development and implementation

- examples of practice guidelines that currently exist on national, state, and local levels
- the concept of outcome measurement, types of outcomes measures, the process of outcome validation, and the importance of outcome-validating guidelines
- examples of disease management programs using an evidence-based approach

TREATMENT AND DIAGNOSTIC OVERUTILIZATION: A HEALTH CARE DILEMMA

Rising costs related to treatment and diagnosis have caused the health care system to come under great scrutiny. In 1996, the U.S. Department of Commerce estimated that the United States will spend approximately $1 trillion on health care.[2] This means that health care represents approximately 14% of the gross domestic product (GDP), compared to 6% in 1965.[2] Additionally, the Congressional Budget Office predicted that by the year 2000, health care expenditures could reach $1.7 trillion, or 18% of the GDP.[3] In an attempt to remedy this situation, investigations have been conducted to identify patterns of medical practice, as well as to specify areas for possible reduction of inappropriate health care.

Variations in patient care were demonstrated in several studies[4-9] (see Exhibit 3–1), possibly identifying overutilization of services in certain instances. One investigation, which tested practice variations, demonstrated that 2500 more hysterectomies were performed over a 10-year period in one Maine community than were performed in a neighboring area of similar demographics and dimensions. With a cost of approximately $4000 for each procedure, the difference could have amounted to an excess of $10 million.[8] Similar rates of variation were demonstrated for tonsillectomies in children. One area had a 70% tonsillectomy rate in children under 15 years of age, whereas another had less than an 8% tonsillectomy rate in a similar population.[8,9] These variations highlighted the need to define better what is appropriate medical care.

PAST ATTEMPTS AT MEDICAL COST CONTAINMENT

Concerns about rising health care costs led to the implementation of many different cost containment strategies that resulted in a number of innovations in the health care system.[10] From an economic standpoint, the physician and hospital reimbursement arrangement began transforming from the characteristic fee-for-service model into an integrated, capitated payment structure. From a health care delivery standpoint, the conventional model of private physician practice or small groups of physician practices began shifting to a managed-care model.[10] The man-

Exhibit 3–1 Medical and Surgical Causes of Admissions, Ranked in Ascending Order of Variation in Incidence of Hospitalization (1980–1982)

Medical Causes of Admission

Low Variation
None

Moderate Variation
Acute myocardial infarction (AMI)
Gastrointestinal hemorrhage
Specific cerebrovascular disorders

High Variation
Nutritional and metabolic diseases
Syncope and collapse
Respiratory neoplasms
Cellulitis
Urinary tract stones
Cardiac arrhythmias
Miscellaneous injuries to extremities
Angina pectoris
Toxic effects of drugs
Psychosis
Heart failure and shock
Seizures and headaches
Adult simple pneumonias
Respiratory signs and symptoms
Depressive neurosis
Medical back problems
Gastrointestinal obstruction
Adult gastroenteritis
Peripheral vascular disorders
Red blood cell disorders
Adult diabetes
Circulatory disorders except AMI
  with cardiac catheter

Very High Variation
Deep-vein thrombophlebitis
Adult bronchitis and asthma
Organic mental syndromes
Chest pain

Transient ischemic attacks
Kidney and urinary tract infections
Acute adjustment reaction
Minor skin disorders
Trauma to skin, subcutaneous tissue, and
  breast
Chronic obstructive lung disease
Hypertension
Adult otitis media and upper respiratory
  infections (URIs)
Peptic ulcer
Disorders of the biliary tract
Pediatric gastroenteritis
Pediatric bronchitis and asthma
Atherosclerosis
Pediatric otitis media and URIs
Pediatric pneumonia

Surgical Causes of Admissions

Low Variation
Inguinal and femoral hernia repair
Hip repair except joint replacement

Moderate Variation
Appendicitis with appendectomy
Major small- and large-bowel surgery
Gall bladder disease with cholecystec-
  tomy
Adult hernia repairs except inguinal and
  femoral

High Variation
Hysterectomy
Major cardiovascular operations
Pediatric hernia operations
Hand operations except ganglion
Foot operations

continues

Exhibit 3–1 continued

Surgical Causes of Admission
Major joint operations
Stomach, esophageal, and duodenal
  operations
Anal operations
Female reproductive system recon-
  structive operations
Back and neck operations
Soft tissue operations

Very High Variation
Knee operations
Transurethral operations
Uterus and andenexa operations

Extraocular operations
Misc. ear, nose, and throat operations
Breast biopsy and local excision for
  nonmalignancy
D&C except for malignancy
T&A operations except for tonsillec-
  tomy
Tonsillectomy
Female laparoscopic operations except
  for sterilization
Dental extractions and restorations
Laparoscopic tubal interruptions
Tubal interruption for nonmalignancy

Note: Causes or hospitalizations are taken from diagnostic-related disease classification system, but cases have been grouped without regard to presence or absence of significant complications. Obstetrical and neonatal causes of hospitalization are excluded. Ranking is according to the systematic component of variation. Variations are measured across 30 hospital markets. The exhibit lists individually only those with more than 1500 cases. More than 50% of hospitalizations are represented in the exhibit. Classes of variation are defined such that the variation associated with the first entry in a class is significantly more variable than the first entry in the previous class. For additional information, see source. *Source:* Reprinted with permission from J.E. Wennberg, Dealing with Medical Practice Variations: A Proposal for Action, *Health Affairs,* Vol. 3, No. 2, p. 14, © 1984, The People to People Health Foundation, Inc.

aged-care movement evolved as an attempt to manage and finance health care delivery to ensure that services provided were necessary and appropriately priced.[11] Various aspects of managed care were then evaluated in an effort to define more clearly how this arrangement was affecting patient care. The RAND Health Insurance Experiment demonstrated that requirements for copayments reduced doctor visits and hospitalizations without a diminution in health outcomes for most patients.[12] Another study showed that health maintenance organization (HMO) patients received fewer services than fee-for-service patients for similar conditions without adverse effects on their health.[13] In the hospital setting, cost containment efforts were specifically focused on reducing inpatient costs.[14] Lengths of stay were shortened; inpatient procedures and tests were reduced.[14] But although this may have resulted in lower inpatient expenses, reduction of costs in the hospital may have been offset by increased costs outside the hospital.[14] In these instances, costs were not being reduced but merely shifted to other settings.[14] As this cost-shifting phenomenon was recognized, it became clear that the cost reduction had to be demonstrated across the health care continuum to evaluate the effects of these initiatives.

THE CONCEPT OF DISEASE MANAGEMENT

Improving care across the continuum is the underlying premise of disease management. Disease management begins with an understanding of the natural history of a disease and a determination of when best to proceed to implement a defined quality improvement or cost reduction program.[15] Disease management often incorporates disease prevention and health promotion and relies on evidence-based treatments using clinical practice guidelines.[16] In essence, these programs may constitute a platform for the clinical care process. Managing patient care may require targeting key steps in the clinical care process. Disease management programs may address these areas, thereby assisting physicians in arriving at the correct diagnosis; ensuring that patients are treated appropriately for the severity of their disease; guiding the course of patients' treatment through valid, scientific clinical practice guidelines; educating patients as well as physicians; and providing case management through the entire course of treatment.[10] Typically, the diagnostic, evaluation, and treatment components constitute the inception of this comprehensive process. The latter portion concerns measuring and tracking patient outcomes. The outcomes measurement process examines whether the program has truly demonstrated real value and identifies opportunities to further modify and improve the patient care process.[10] This should be a data-driven process that is capable of being rapidly translated to provide clinical insight into the best practices for patient care.[16]

PHYSICIANS' PERSPECTIVE ON DISEASE MANAGEMENT

To date, we know of no studies evaluating physicians' attitudes about disease management. However, our experience has led us to believe that the physician's primary concern is how the disease management program affects the quality of patients' care. When disease management programs are based on scientific studies that have demonstrated that a particular approach has in fact improved the quality of care, physicians tend to be encouraged about the approach's use. Physicians also tend to be extremely concerned with maintaining, if not improving, patient satisfaction. Therefore, the impact of the program on patient satisfaction and continuity of care is a prime concern. Additionally, physicians may look favorably upon a disease management program if the program reduces the routine work and allows them to spend more time with patients or diagnosing and treating more perplexing medical problems.

When considering a disease management program, physicians may become concerned if a program does not demonstrate an improvement in patient care and if the program disrupts the continuity of care. Physicians may also stop supporting a program if the time spent complying with the administrative work takes away from time that they should spend with their patients.

CLINICAL PRACTICE GUIDELINES

History

Practice guidelines provide a foundation of the scientific evidence for disease management programs. However, the concept of clinical practice guidelines is not a recent innovation. For many years, groups have developed and used guidelines for different purposes: as educational tools for physicians in training, as a reference to resolve clinical controversies, as a way to control costs, as an attempt to reduce variation in treatment patterns, and as an attempt to improve medical outcomes.[17] But although guidelines have been available for decades, their adoption has been relatively limited.

Over the past few decades, many public and private organizations have been actively developing guidelines. The federal government sponsors guideline development through organizations such as Agency for Health Care Policy and Research (AHCPR), the National Institutes of Health (NIH), the Centers for Disease Control and Prevention (CDC), and the U.S. Preventative Services Task Force (USPSTF).[18] Additionally, private organizations (eg, the American Medical Association), medical specialty societies (eg, American College of Cardiology, American Heart Association), and private research organizations (eg, The RAND Corporation) have participated in guidelines efforts.[18] As the movement has progressed, with national organizations actively developing guidelines, some local organizations have begun to develop more guidelines that they have considered more relevant at the local level.[19]

Development

The guideline development process is summarized in Exhibit 3–2. It begins with identification of specific clinical conditions that may be more appropriately managed through a more regulated approach. Typically, these tend to be the conditions that are the most common and the most costly and that have demonstrated a substantial amount of variation in clinician treatment patterns (eg, diabetes, hypertension). By targeting the areas that meet the previously mentioned criteria, an institution may maximize return on investment and minimize expended resources.

Exhibit 3–2 Development of Evidence-Based Guidelines

Step 1: Identify a clinical condition.
Step 2: Review scientific literature.
Step 3: Translate guidelines into "executable statements."
Step 4: Obtain physician acceptance.
Step 5: Compare guideline with current practice.
Step 6: Develop a system to identify eligible patients.
Step 7: Educate health care providers and patients.
Step 8: Implement guidelines.
Step 9: Evaluate effectiveness of guideline implementation.
Step 10: Assess the effects of the guideline on patient care.
Step 11: Improve the guideline.

Once the institution has identified target areas requiring improvement, the next step involves reviewing the scientific literature. This procedure ultimately creates the structural support for the guideline. Various evidentiary grading scales have been proposed. We have used an adaptation of the Evidence-Based Medicine Group at McMaster University (Exhibit 3–3).[20] This grading scale classifies the articles according to their study design. Once the literature is categorized, summarized, and graded, the evidence should be evaluated by clinical research experts.

Once the literature has been deemed relevant and of sufficient scientific rigor to assist with medical decision making, the guideline should be translated into "executable statements." The statements could read as "if, then"–type expressions. For example, one chest pain guideline reads, "If the patient does not have a myocardial infarction, recurrent chest pain, unstable comorbidity, prior, ongoing, or planned intervention, then the physician should consider discharging the patient after 48 hours."[21] Additionally, statements should be written so that they can be interpreted consistently from one user to the next. In other words, after reading the guideline, each practitioner should have received the same message as the next practitioner. An example of a guideline that is *not* executable is "Transfer patient out of intensive care unit when stable." This statement is vague and leaves a great deal of interpretation to the practitioner, which may ultimately result in variations in practice.

Subsequently, the proposed guideline should be tested and compared to current practice in an attempt to be certain that any deviation from "care as usual" will truly benefit the patient. This step has in several cases been accomplished through an observational or retrospective study design in which a guideline can be tested to determine how care may have differed from care provided before the guideline

Exhibit 3–3 Grades of Evidence

Grade A Recommendation
⇨ Randomized, prospective, controlled trials

Grade B Recommendation
⇨ Nonrandomized, prospective, controlled trials

Grade C Recommendation
⇨ Any retrospective analysis

Grade E Recommendation
⇨ Information based on indirect evidence, personal experience, or expert opinion

Grade M Recommendation
⇨ Supported by at least one meta-analysis

Grade Q Recommendation
⇨ Supported by at least one cost-effectiveness or decision analysis

Grade S Recommendation
⇨ Supported by at least ony study that summarizes and pools data from other articles

---

was implemented in that particular patient population.[22,23] During this evaluation process, it is also advantageous to confirm that the proposed guideline addresses the continuum of care in order to avoid "cost shifting."

Before implementing the guideline, one should attempt to obtain physician "buy-in." If physicians do not trust the guideline development process, then they may not use the guideline.[24] This is one of the reasons that the evidence-based approach along with expert opinion may be more successful than the expert opinion approach unsupported by scientific evidence. Physicians often trust scientific evidence, whereas expert opinion is more subjectively based. To accomplish this undertaking, provider involvement should occur. First, health care providers should be educated on the contents and scientific foundation of the guideline and encouraged to contribute their expertise to promote physician acceptance. Once this is accomplished, the guideline implementation process may begin.

Implementation

Practice guideline dissemination efforts often begin with continuing medical education.[25] It was once thought that education as a means to disseminate guidelines would be a relatively cost-effective method of disseminating clinical information to physicians and other clinicians across the country. But although the concept was promising, it was largely unsuccessful.[26] Millions of dollars later, continuing medical education efforts as a means of disseminating guidelines have yet to provide a significant and sustainable impact on improving quality of patient care and patient outcomes or on sustaining long-term changes in clinical practice.[25, 27-29] Distinguished national organizations have also participated in efforts to disseminate practice guidelines. For example, in the late 1970s, NIH created a program called the Consensus Development Program that was charged with keeping physicians and other health care providers informed of the latest technological breakthroughs.[30] The assumption was that published guidelines developed by world-renowned medical experts would cause physicians to incorporate them into their own practices. However, this assumption also proved to be incorrect. Although some physicians were aware of these recommendations, their practice often did not change to conform to the guidelines.[30] Implementation efforts involving a combination of strategies, rather than education alone, have proven to be more effective.

Successful methods of implementation may be institution specific. Cedars-Sinai Health System, in Los Angeles, California, has had some success with intensive education, followed by concurrent reminders to prompt practitioners regarding guideline contents in real time[31] (see Exhibit 3–4). Studies have shown that constant intervention is required in order to change physician practices because education alone is insufficient.[21,32-34] In a chest pain guideline, Cedars-Sinai Health System utilized a combination of education, physician participation in guideline development, and concurrent and written feedback.[21] These interventions resulted in a 19% increase in compliance with the guideline, as compared with attempts before continuous intervention.[21] This increase demonstrated a relationship between the continuous reminders and an increase in physician compliance with the guideline. A second study was conducted to analyze reasons for

---

Exhibit 3–4 Potential Methods To Increase Physician Compliance with Guidelines

- Concurrent feedback
- Retrospective feedback
- "Academic detailing"
- Opinion leaders
- Case management
- Disease management clinic
- Incentives
- Removal of disincentives
- Information technology
  (reminders and warnings)

Source: © *Journal of Quality Improvement.* Oakbrook Terrace, IL: Joint Commission on Accreditation of Healthcare Organizations, 1996, p. 562. Reprinted with permission.

noncompliance with the chest pain guideline in an attempt to further improve physician compliance. The study concluded that only 16% of total noncompliance was due to physician refusal, whereas the greater part of noncompliance was due to implementation issues, health care system inefficiencies, and severity of patient illness[35] (see Figure 3–1).

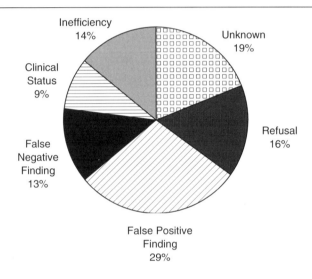

Unknown:
No apparent resons found on retrospective chart review

Refusal:
Physician Refusal

False Positive Finding:
Patients misclassified as being low-risk when they were actually considered high-risk

False Negative Finding:
1. Patients misclassified as being high-risk, and therefore were not contacted
2. Patients not enrolled in the study despite meeting eligibility requirements

Clinical Status:
Change in clinical status between 24 and 48 hours

Inefficiency:
Health Care Inefficiency: Physicians agrees to discharge patients on day 2, but the system held them until day 3

Figure 3–1 Reasons for Not Following a Chest Pain Guideline. Source: *Journal of Quality Improvement.* Oakbrook Terrace, IL: Joint Commission on Accreditation of Healthcare Organizations, 1996, p. 563. Reprinted with permission.

Practice Guidelines Currently in Existence

National Level

Currently, multiple guidelines are being developed and used on a national level. There have been significant successes with practice guidelines that have led to better patient care. For example, in the past, indications for pacemakers varied considerably, resulting in many people receiving pacemakers for what might be categorized as inappropriate indications. In the 1980s, the American College of Cardiology developed a guideline addressing the appropriate utilization of cardiac pacemakers.[36] The development of this guideline was a response to the perceived overutilization of implantable cardiac pacemakers. A task force was assigned the responsibility of defining the indications for permanent cardiac pacemakers, as well as recommendations regarding the appropriate selection of devices for the specific clinical conditions for which the pacemaker was indicated.[36] Once these guidelines were widely disseminated to physicians, utilization rates for pacemakers declined significantly (see Figure 3–2).[36,37]

Another example is a result of the work of the American Society of Anesthesiologists (ASA). In 1968, the ASA published its first set of guidelines.[38] These were standards that were based on the recommendations of a committee that represented nine hospitals affiliated with Harvard University.[38,39] They were "Standards for Basic Intraoperative Monitoring," intended to focus on risk management activities for clinical practices that gave rise to the greatest number of malpractice claims.[39–42] During the decade ending in December 1986, the Massachusetts Medical Malpractice Joint Underwriting Association (JUA), the only insurance company available for the majority of anesthesiologists practicing in Massachusetts, had 27 closed claims involving hypoxic injury.[42,43] In 1987, JUA offered a 20% premium discount on liability insurance to all anesthesiologists who agreed to abide by the practice guideline.[42,43] The Massachusetts physicians' hypoxic injury lawsuit rate went from 6% per year before the guideline was implemented to no hypoxic injury lawsuits the following year among those who followed the guideline.[42,43]

Not all attempts to implement guidelines are successful. For instance, asthma guidelines were developed by the Expert Panel on the Management of Asthma assembled by the National Asthma Education Program and supported by the National Heart, Lung, and Blood Institute of NIH, for the diagnosis and management of asthma.[44] After the guidelines were distributed to family physicians, family physicians decided that these guidelines might be inappropriate for use by family physicians for the following three reasons: lack of family physician representation on the guideline development panel, the panel's subjective development process, and failure to base the guidelines on the basic science underlying asthma diagnosis and treatment.[24] Although the developers were respected and from prestigious or-

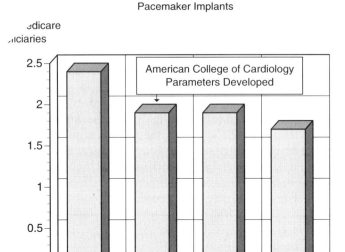

Figure 3–2 Effects of Guidelines on Rate of Inappropriate Performance of a Procedure. Since the implementation of the 1984 American College of Cardiology practice parameters for pacemaker implants, utilization rates for pacemakers among Medicare patients have significantly declined. *Source:* Reprinted with permission from J.B. Mitchell, G. Wedig, and J. Cromwell, The Medicare Physician Fee Freeze: What Really Happened?, *Health Affairs,* Vol. 8, No. 1, p. 27, © 1989, The People To People Health Foundation, Inc.

ganizations, guidelines that were based on expert opinion rather than scientific evidence were not adopted.[24]

State Level

Statewide guideline efforts range from Maine to Rhode Island and Wisconsin, where the impact that guidelines may have as a cost containment and tort reform mechanism is being studied.[45–49] Some states have introduced guidelines to offer protection in malpractice cases as an affirmative defense. The state of Maine, for example, has pioneered the use of guidelines as an affirmative defense with their 5-year Liability Demonstration Project,[45–48] which was enacted in 1990 and amended in 1992. The goal of the Maine project is to limit health care cost increases by offering protection from malpractice suits when physicians comply with the guidelines. Specifically, the law provides protection for physicians in four high-risk specialties (anesthesiology, obstetrics/gynecology, radiology, and emergency medicine).[45-49] The premise is that if physicians are protected when they comply with the guidelines, then there will be a decrease in defensive medical procedures, which have been proposed as a major contributor to health care costs. As Maine law currently stands, only the physician or the physician's employer may introduce clinical practice guidelines as an affirmative defense when charged with professional negligence. Guidelines cannot be used by the plaintiff's attorney against physicians who fail to comply with the guidelines.[45-47] As one might have suspected, this concept has instigated a substantial amount of debate between the medical and legal communities.[49-52]

Another example of a state's approach to using guidelines involves Caesarean sections. During the last 20 years, Caesarean section rates have quadrupled from 5.5% in 1970 to 22% in 1990 in the United States.[53] This has been a great concern because Caesarean sections result in more patient discomfort following delivery and are more costly procedures than vaginal deliveries. In an attempt to decrease costs, hospitals were discharging mothers and their babies 24 hours after vaginal delivery. Due to public concern, legislation was passed on a national level that mandated a minimum 48-hour postpartum stay in the hospital for patients who delivered vaginally unless a doctor overruled this suggestion.[54] However, Florida took a different approach to rectify this problem. The state of Florida's Committee on Maternal and Newborn Hospital Discharge Guidelines, endorsed by the Agency for Health Care Administration (AHCA), pursuant to the Florida Health Care and Insurance Reform Act of 1993, identified the typical criteria for discharging mothers and their newborns following delivery.[55] They developed hospital discharge criteria in which *early discharge* meant 24 to 48 hours and *very early discharge* meant less than 24 hours. The guideline was developed to remedy concerns about early maternal and newborn discharge by more clearly defining who could and who could not be discharged from the hospital safely.[55]

Local Level

Contributions to guideline development and implementation have been made at a number of institutions. At Cedars-Sinai Medical Center, in Los Angeles, California, we believe that the use of evidence-based medicine to develop guidelines will lead to greatest physician acceptance of practice guidelines.[56] At Cedars-Sinai, guidelines are developed using the evidence-based process through integration of the latest scientific literature combined with clinical expertise. One of Cedars-Sinai's most thoroughly evaluated guidelines was a chest pain guideline that resulted in early discharge of patients who had been initially hospitalized with chest pain (see Figure 3–3).[32] The guideline was initially developed through an examination of the scientific literature. Once it was developed, an observational study was done to test it and determine what would happen if it was implemented.[22] Then the guideline was used in a controlled trial with an alternate-month

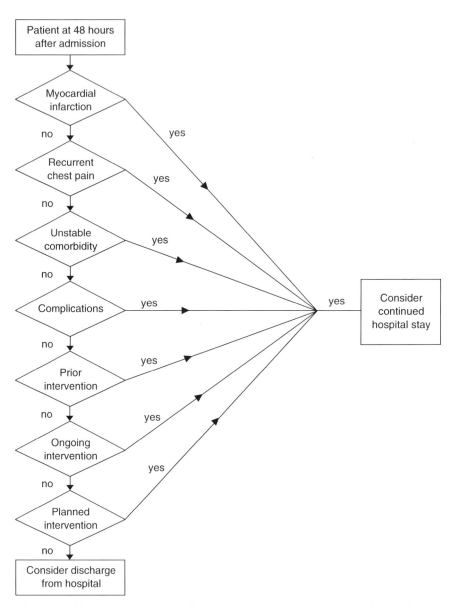

Figure 3–3 Cedar-Sinai Chest Pain Guideline. Patients without myocardial infarction, recurrent chest pain, unstable comorbidity, complications, a previous major intervention, an ongoing intervention requiring care in the coronary care unit, or a planned coronary care unit intervention were considered potentially suitable for discharge from the hospital after 48 hours. Otherwise, continued hospitalization was considered potentially appropriate. *Source:* Reprinted with permission from S. Weingarten, et al., Early "Step Down" Transfer of Low-Risk Patients with Chest Pain, *Annals of Internal Medicine,* Vol. 113, pp. 283–289, © 1990, American College of Physicians.

study design. The intervention was a phone call to the physicians caring for "low-risk" patients in the coronary care unit and intensive care unit 24 hours after patient admission. Physicians were contacted and informed that the transfer of low-risk patients could probably be done safely, and the risk of complications was communicated.[32] The effects of this effort to disseminate guidelines were encouraging. There were no distinguishable differences between patients who were discharged early and patients with longer lengths of stay, except that the early discharge guideline was saving an average of $1400 per low-risk patient (indirect and direct costs). At Cedars-Sinai, this intervention saved the hospital approximately $500,000 per year. The cost of the guideline development was between $50,000 and $100,000, with an annual operating cost of $30,000.[21,57] Moreover, outcomes including quality of care and complication rates demonstrated no significant differences.

A similar type of guideline was developed at Cedars-Sinai Medical Center for patients with congestive heart failure.[58] Patients were classified as low risk or high risk to determine whether they could be safely transferred to a nonmonitored bed 24 hours after admission. The premise behind decreasing the coronary care unit (CCU) length of stay was based on literature suggesting that matching each patient's condition to the most appropriate level of care would increase CCU and intensive care unit (ICU) bed availability,[59] reduce unnecessarily prolonged lengths of stay, and improve the quality of patient care.[60–64] The guideline was first assessed using a hypothetical experimental design. Data collection was obtained through medical records to determine whether each patient was considered low risk or high risk on the basis of a practice guideline that was approved by 150 ICU directors in the state of Massachussetts,[65] and then modified by a panel of six physicians at Cedars-Sinai Medical Center.[58] According to the guideline, of the patients that were classified as low risk, 98% survived hospitalization, whereas 2% were transferred to another hospital. In comparison, of the patients classified as high risk, 82% survived hospitalization, whereas 6% were transferred to another hospital.[58] From this hypothetical study, it was concluded that the early step-down transfer of the low-risk patients with congestive heart failure had a significant potential to improve bed availability in the CCU and ICU while reducing expenditures. However, before recommending the guideline for widespread use, the team at Cedars-Sinai did a prospective, controlled trial with an alternate-month study design.[65] The intervention in this trial consisted of verbal and written reminders of the guideline recommendation to the physicians caring for low-risk patients. The results, contrary to the hypothetical experiment, demonstrated not only that there was no significant reduction in monitored bed lengths of stay but that total length of stay actually increased after the guideline was implemented. The complexity of the guideline and its failure to address the continuum of care across monitored and unmonitored beds may have accounted for these findings. Additionally, physician compliance with the guideline, using techniques that had been proven effective in the past,[21,32,66] was limited. This experience demonstrated the importance of validating guidelines through testing and measuring patient outcomes. The lesson is that although guidelines may be based on reputable sources and may appear promising, it is crucial that they address the continuum of care and be evaluated in clinical practice before they are recommended for widespread use.[65]

OUTCOME MEASUREMENT

The Premise behind Measuring Outcomes

Though guidelines are responsible for guiding patient care, tracking the end results of guidelines to verify that care has actually improved is important. Outcome measurement is a process used to determine whether the recommendations of practice guidelines do, in fact, optimize patient care. The outcome validation process should serve as a means of isolating the most effective processes, which may ultimately contribute to increased physician comfort with and acceptance of guidelines, not to mention improved patient health.

More specifically, outcome measurement serves as a means of establishing effectiveness of patient care in the "real-world" setting.[67] These types of results provide practitioners with the appropriate information with which to identify what does and does not work when treating their patients.[67] In other words, the results of outcome measurement can be used to assess the quality of the care that the caregiver is providing his or her patients. In essence, these quality measures can be used internally for quality improvement purposes or externally as indicators for comparison of the quality of care delivered among multiple care providers and health care organizations (e.g., the Health Care Financing Administration's release of physician and hospital mortality statistics,[20] or Health Plan Employer Data and Information Set [HEDIS] indicators).

Types of Outcome Measures

Outcomes are typically categorized as *clinical outcomes* (e.g., myocardial infarction, death), *economic outcomes* (e.g., direct cost of hospitalizations), or *patient-centered outcomes* (quality of life, patient satisfaction).[16] Which outcomes are measured tends to be a result of the focus of those examining the data or the perspective from which the data are analyzed. For instance, patients may be most interested in patient-centered outcomes (quality of life), and clinicians have traditionally been interested in clinical outcomes, but increasingly many parties have become interested in economic and patient-centered outcomes.[16] To measure the various outcomes available, a multitude of instruments have been developed and studied. Typically, these instruments consist of a series of specific questions that have been tested and confirmed to determine certain specific outcome measures regarding the patient's health status. Some instruments are developed as generic instruments that may be transportable among patients with different disease states (e.g., the Medical Outcomes Study's SF-36, a validated instrument for measuring overall health status), whereas other instruments have been developed to be disease specific (eg, the Inflammatory Bowel Disease Quality of Life Questionnaire or the Kidney Transplant Recipient Stress Scale). These instruments are assessed using psychometric evaluation procedures to determine whether each tool is reliable, responsive, and valid.[68]

It is important to have a clear understanding of a true outcome versus an intermediate outcome or process measure. A true outcome measure should demonstrate whether the intended results of the patient's care processes have been achieved. For example, the outcome is not defined as an increase in mammography screening rates but as how many clinical complications were prevented or detected, or how many lives were saved. In this example, the mammography screening would represent an intermediate outcome or process measure, whereas the number of clinical complications prevented might represent a true outcome. For post–hip replacement procedures, the number of hip replacement patients put on deep-venous thrombosis prophylaxis might be the intermediate outcome (or process measure), but the number of patients who did not develop a deep-venous thrombosis might be the true outcome. Outcome measure types are summarized in Exhibit 3–5.

The Outcome Validation Process

The outcome validation process, summarized in Exhibit 3–6, starts with the appropriate selection of process measures. Although a specific list of process

---

Exhibit 3–5 Outcome Measure Categories

Clinical outcomes
  • Intermediate outcome or process measure (e.g., mammography screening rate)
  • True outcome measure (e.g., clinical complications prevented)
Economic outcomes
  • Direct costs (e.g., cost of hospitalization)
  • Indirect costs (e.g., days of work lost)
Patient-centered outcomes
  • Quality of life
  • Health status
  • Patient satisfaction

Source: Reprinted with permission from Epstein and Sherwood, Outcomes Research to Disease Management: A Guide for the Perplexed, *Annals of Internal Medicine,* Vol. 124, pp. 832–837, © 1996, American College of Physicians.

Exhibit 3–6 The Outcome Validation Process

Step 1:	Select appropriate process measures.
Step 2:	Select appropriate outcome measures.
Step 3:	Determine method of data collection.
Step 4:	Determine appropriate timing of data collection.
Step 5:	Determine cost of data collection.
Step 6:	Analyze the data.

measures has not been created, specific criteria of process measures were identified by Paul Lembcke[69] in 1956. Lembcke's process measure criteria include the following:

- *Objectivity.* The criteria should be developed with appropriate precision and detail to minimize any variability in interpretation (e.g., "Patients who meet the following criteria are considered low-risk patients").
- *Verifiability.* The criteria should be based on points that can be documented and confirmed by the patient's medical record (e.g., laboratory tests, specific diagnoses that should be documented in the chart).
- *Uniformity.* Criteria should be developed independent of factors such as hospital size or location, qualifications of the physician, or socioeconomic status of the patient population.
- *Specificity.* Criteria should be specific for each specific disease or operation (eg, hypertension process measure—blood pressure measurements; hip replacement process measure—deep-venous thrombosis prophylaxis).
- *Pertinence.* Criteria should be pertinent to the ultimate goal of care, with specific consideration of results rather than intentions (eg, this process has been studied and should relate to changes in outcomes).
- *Acceptability.* Criteria should conform to generally accepted standards of good quality.

After process measures have been elucidated, the next step is to select appropriate outcome measures. The various types of outcomes have been mentioned on page 72. However, when selecting the specific outcome measures, one should also consider the same criteria as for the process measures. For example, for total hip replacement, outcome measures might include survival, postoperative infection rate, deep-venous thrombosis rate, reoperation rate, length of stay, cost, discharge location, readmission rate, return to emergency department, health status/quality of life, patient satisfaction, return to work, and ability to return home and resume recreational activities. Once the appropriate process and outcome measures have been selected, the next step involves determination of the best and most cost-effective methods of collecting this information (eg, patient surveys, chart review, administrative databases). Factors that may be considered when determining the best method of information collection at each institution may include the databases to which each institution has access, the reliability and validity of the information, and the cost of data collection. Once the data collection method and the collection of data have been completed, the next step in the process is to analyze the data.

The Importance of Outcome-Validated Guidelines

As the clinical practice guideline movement continues to flourish, the medical establishment will continue to look for more innovative ways of using guidelines to benefit patients and the health care system. Meanwhile, the guidelines that are currently being developed should be tested to ensure that they will improve the practice of medicine. This testing process has been called outcome validation (see Figure 3–4). The effect of the intervention should be explicitly linked to the outcomes that the guideline is supposed to improve.[70] Using an outcome-based approach, the developers of the guideline should define the interventions, the intended outcomes, and the evidence that demonstrates that the intervention

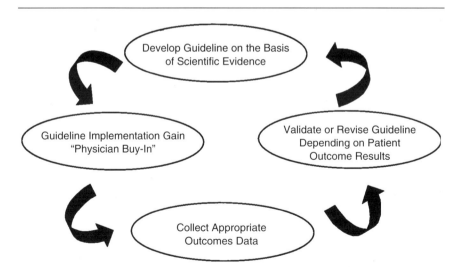

Figure 3–4 Outcome Validation of Guidelines: A Continuous Improvement Process

produces improvements in the desired outcome.[70] In the past, measurement of dichotomous outcomes such as survival or occurrence of a clinical event was often performed. At the present time, measures such as patient satisfaction, quality of life, and functional status are being reported with increasing frequency.[16]

The outcome validation process can benefit the multiple stakeholders involved in guideline development. For instance, providers may benefit by using outcomes assessment to select the best guidelines for their patients. Payers may benefit by reforming the decision-making process that determines which treatments merit reimbursement. Patients may benefit from improvements in quality of care.[67]

Health care providers are faced with multiple issues by public and private payers. Hospitals and other health care organizations may use outcome-validated results to develop and implement clinical practice guidelines at the local level and to identify areas for quality improvement. Payers may use outcome-validated guidelines to identify areas of ineffective care, with the hope of eliminating unnecessary medical procedures and treatments; to determine which services to reimburse; or to establish a foundation from which to select the highest-quality health care providers (eg, HEDIS).[67]

RECENT DISEASE MANAGEMENT PROGRAMS USING AN EVIDENCE-BASED APPROACH TO GUIDELINES

Although clinical practice guidelines were used at Cedars-Sinai Health System in Los Angeles, California, about a decade ago, disease management efforts commenced in 1995. Programs were developed using an evidence-based approach. Each program includes clinical recommendations based on the scientific literature combined with clinician expertise, considers the use of physician extenders in addition to physicians to further enhance patient care, emphasizes patient education, measures specified patient outcomes, and addresses the continuum of patient care.

The first program developed was a Hypertension Disease Management Program, which has been implemented at the Cedars-Sinai Medical Care Foundation's Medical Group of Beverly Hills by Drs. Jeff Borenstein, Geneen Graber, Steve Deutsch, Tina Thai, and Emanuel Saltiel. Hypertension was selected due to its high prevalence, significant long-term morbidity, mortality, and high cost. The program includes a drug protocol initially based on the recently published Joint National Committee on Hypertension V recommendations[71] (see Figure 3–5). It involves a hypertension clinic that is managed by a clinical pharmacist and supervised by physicians. The pharmacist visit includes blood pressure measurements and patient education relaying medical, dietary, and medication-related information. All therapeutic changes, based on the drug protocol, require patient, study pharmacist, and primary care physician approval. Specified outcomes are tracked and assessed. These include clinical outcomes (blood pressure control), patient-

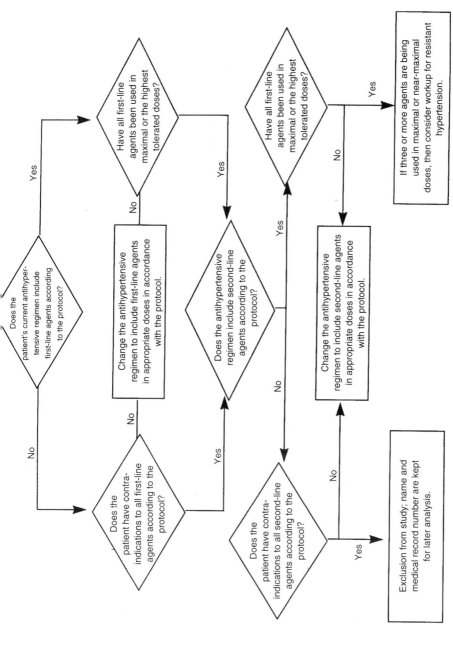

Figure 3–5 Cedars-Sinai Hypertension Clinic Pharmacologic Protocol. Courtesy of Cedars-Sinai Health System, Beverly Hills, California.

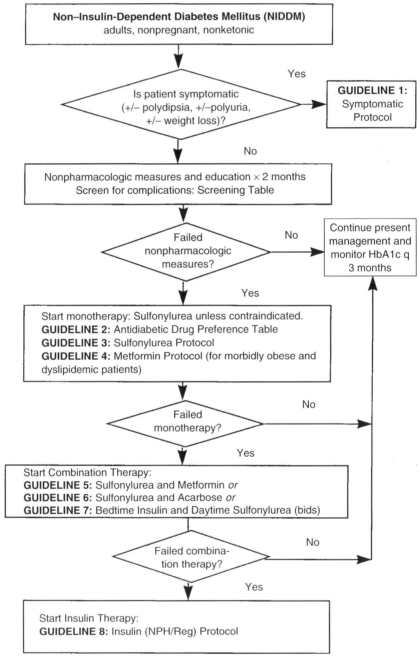

Figure 3–6 Cedars-Sinai Non–Insulin-Dependent Diabetes Mellitus Guideline. Courtesy of Cedars-Sinai Health System, Beverly Hills, California.

centered outcomes (health status and symptomatology), and economic outcomes (medication, lab, and visit costs). Through patient counseling, lifestyle modifications, evidence-based therapeutic recommendations, and the measurement of specified patient outcomes, this program is intended to improve overall patient health status by addressing the continuum of care while using a cost-effective approach.

Another project is a diabetes disease management program. This project is led by Drs. Jean Lee, Michael Harris, Steve Deutsch, and Katie Arce. Diabetes mellitus is also an ideal condition for application of the principles of disease management, since improvements in health outcomes have been researched. For example, the Diabetes Control and Complications Trial (DCCT) was a multicenter, randomized, controlled clinical trial that demonstrated a significant delay in onset and progression of diabetic retinopathy, nephropathy, and neuropathy with intensive insulin therapy compared to conventional therapy in insulin-dependent diabetes mellitus patients.[72] Thus, there is strong supporting evidence to normalize blood glucose concentrations to prevent the onset and slow the progression of long-term complications.[73,74] Interventions such as these with a process and outcome link have been translated into clinical guidelines that are implemented in a Diabetes Center at Cedars-Sinai Medical Care Foundation (see Figure 3–6). The effectiveness of the clinical guidelines will be measured by analyzing their associated clinical (glycosylated hemoglobin, rate of retinal exams), patient-centered (health status and symptomatology), and economic outcomes (rate of work absenteeism). These outcome measurements can then be translated into feedback strategies to make improvements in patient quality of care on a continuous basis.

America's health care system is moving toward a disease management model.[75] The most promising programs may include the use of practice guidelines. However, to make certain that each patient's quality of care is not compromised and is in fact improved, the guidelines must be based on scientific data. Evidence-based medical care and the use of outcomes-based practice guidelines are bringing us closer to the solution of providing high-quality, cost-effective medical care.

References

1. American Medical Association. *Directory of Practice Parameters.* Chicago, Ill: AMA; 1996.

2. US Dept. of Commerce. *Health Care Expenditures.* Washington, DC: US Dept of Commerce; 1996.

3. US Congress, Congressional Budget Office. *Economic Implications of Rising Health Care Costs.* Washington, DC; 1992.

4. Wennberg JE. The need for assessing the outcome of common medical practices. *Ann Rev Public Health.* 1980;1:277–295.

5. Wennberg JE. Variations in medical practice and hospital costs. *Conn Med.* 1985;49:444–453.

6. Wennberg JE, Gittelsohn A. Variations in medical care among small areas. *Sci Am.* 1982; 246:120–134.

7. Wennberg JE, Gittelsohn A. Small area variations in health care delivery. *Science.* 1973; 142:1102–1108.

8. Wennberg JE. Dealing with medical practice variations: a proposal for action. *Health Aff.* 1984; 3:6–32.

9. Wennberg JE, et al. Changes in tonsillectomy rates associated with feedback and review. *Pediatrics.* 1977;59:821–826.

10. Dubois RW, et al. Disease management: the maturation and application of health services research. *Compensation Benefits Manage.* 1995;11(3):20–30.

11. Fazen M. *Managed Care Desk Reference.* HCS Publications; 1994.

12. Lohr KN, et al. *Use of Medical Care in the RAND Health Insurance Experiment.* Santa Monica, Calif: RAND Corporation; 1986. Publication No. R-3469-HHS.

13. Dorsey JL. Use of diagnostic resources in health maintenance organizations and fee-for-service practice settings. *Arch Intern Med.* 1983;143:1863–1865.

14. Welch HG, et al. The use of Medicare home health care services. *N Eng J Med.* 1996;335:324–329.

15. Boston Consulting Group. *The promise of disease management: the future of health care.* 1995:1–32.

16. Epstein RS, et al. From outcomes research to disease management: a guide for the perplexed. *Ann Intern Med.* 1996;124:832–837.

17. Redman B. Clinical practice guidelines as tools of public policy: conflicts of purpose, issues of autonomy, and justice. *J Clin Ethics.* 1994;5:303–309.

18. US General Accounting Office and HEHS. *Practice Guidelines: Managed Care Plans Customize Guidelines To Meet Local Interest.* Washington, DC; 1996.

19. American Medical Association. *Directory of Practice Parameters.* Chicago, Ill: AMA; 1992.

20. Cook DJ, et al. Rules of evidence and clinical recommendations on the use of antithrombotic agents. *Chest.* 1992;102(suppl.):305S–311S.

21. Weingarten S, et al. Practice guidelines and reminders to reduce duration of hospital stay for patients with chest pain: an interventional trial. *Ann Intern Med.* 1994;120:257.

22. Weingarten S, et al. Selecting the best triage rule for patients hospitalized with chest pain. *Am J Med.* 1988;87:494–500.

23. Weingarten S, et al. Hip replacement and hip hemiarthroplasty surgery: potential opportunities to shorten lengths of hospital stay. *Am J Med.* 1994;97:208–213.

24. Kibbe D, et al. Integrating guidelines with continuous quality improvement: doing the right thing the right way to achieve the right goals. *J Qual Improvement.* 1994;20:181–191.

25. Haynes RB, et al. A critical appraisal of the efficacy of continuing medical education. *JAMA.* 1984;251:61–64.

26. Weingarten SR, Ellrodt AG. The case for intensive dissemination: adoption of practice guidelines in the coronary care unit. *Qual Rev Bull.* December 1992:449–455.

27. Miller LA. The current investment in continuing medical education. In: Egdhal RH, Gertmen PM, eds. *Quality Health Care: The Role of Continuing Medical Education.* Germantown, Md: Aspen Publishers, Inc.: 1977:143–160.

28. Evans CE, et al. Does a mailed continuing education program improve physician performance? Results of a randomized trial in antihypertensive care. *JAMA.* 1986;255:501–504.

29. Sibley JC, et al. A randomized trial of continuing medical education. *N Engl J Med.* 1982; 306:511–515.

30. Kosecoff J, et al. Effects of the National Institutes of Health Consensus Development Program on physician practice. *JAMA.* 1987;258:2708–2713.

31. Weingarten S, et al. Reducing lengths of stay for patients hospitalized with chest pain using medical practice guidelines and opinion leaders. *Am J Cardiol.* 1993;71:259.

32. Weingarten S, et al. Early "step-down" transfer of low-risk patients with chest pain: a controlled interventional trial. *Ann Intern Med.* 1990;113:283–289.

33. Lomas J, et al. Do practice guidelines guide practice? The effect of a consensus statement on the practice of physicians. *N Engl J Med.* 1989;321:1306–1311.

34. Eagle KA, et al. Length of stay in the intensive care unit: effects of practice guidelines and feedback. *JAMA.* 1990;264:992–997.

35. Ellrodt AG, et al. Measuring and improving physician compliance with clinical practice guidelines. *Ann Intern Med.* 1995;122:277–282.

36. Guidelines for permanent cardiac pacemaker implantation: a report of the Joint American College of Cardiology/ American Heart Association Task Force on Assessment of Cardiovascular Procedures. (Subcommittee on Pacemaker Implantation). *J Am Coll Cardiol.* 1982;4:434–442.

37. Pacemakers. *Health Aff.* 1989;8:21–23.

38. American Society of Anesthesiologists. *Annual Directory of Members.* Park Ridge, Ill: ASA; 1968.

39. American Society of Anesthesiologists. *Annual Directory of Members.* Park Ridge, Ill: ASA; 1989.

40. Eichhorn JH, et al. Standards for patient monitoring during anesthesia at Harvard Medical School. *JAMA.* 1986;256:1017–1020.

41. Eichhorn JH, et al. Prevention of intraoperative anesthesia accidents and related severe injury through safety monitoring. *Anesthesiology.* 1989;70:572–577.

42. Pierce E. The development of anesthesia guidelines and standards. *Qual Rev Bull.* February 1990:61–64.

43. Kelly JT, Swartwout JE. Development of practice parameters by physician organizations. *Qual Rev Bull.* Fenruary 1990:54–55.

44. Berg AO, May JG. Guidelines for the diagnosis and management of asthma. *J Am Board Fam Prac.* 1992;5:629–634.

45. US General Accounting Office. *Medical Malpractice: Maine's Use of Practice Guidelines To Reduce Costs.* Gaithersburg, Md.: US GAO; 1993.

46. State of Maine. An Act Concerning Extension of the Notice of Claim Period and Inclusion of Affirmative Defense Consideration in Medical Malpractice Proceedings. 1991. H.P. 943-L.D. 1365.

47. State of Maine. An Act To Include Radiology in the Medical Liability Demonstration Project. 1991. S.P. 495-L.D. 1333.

48. Szabo, J. Practice guidelines: states lay the groundwork. *State Health Notes.* January 1995:4–5.

49. US General Accounting Office. *Medical Malpractice: Alternatives to Litigation.* Gaithersburg, Md.: US GAO; 1992.

50. Hall MA, Dadakis S. Character of guidelines evolves, concern lingers over protection. *Med Malpract: Law Strategy.* 1996;8(4):1–4.

51. Hyams A, et al. Medical practice guidelines in malpractice litigation: an early retrospective. *J Health Politics Policy Law.* 1996;21:288–313.

52. Hirschfeld EB. Should ethical and legal standards for physicians be changed to accomodate new models for rationing health care? *Univ Penn Law Rev.* 1992;140:1809.

53. US Dept of Health and Human Services. *High Malpractice Insurance Premiums Linked with Increased Probability of C-Sections.* Washington, DC: DHHS; 1993. Research Activities No. 162.

54. US General Accounting Office. *Maternity Care: Appropriate Follow-up Services Critical with Short Hospital Stays*. Gaithersburg, Md.: US GAO; 1996.

55. State of Florida. Agency for Health Care Administration. *Postpartum Care of Mothers and Their Newborn Infants Delivered in the Hospital Setting: Medical Malpractice Guidelines*. 1996.

56. Greengold N, Weingarten SR. Developing evidence-based practice guidelines and pathways: the experience at the local hospital level. *J Qual Improvement*. 1996;22:391–402.

57. Leavenworth G. Case studies. Special Report on Guidelines: How Quality Costs Less. *Business and Health*. 12:supp B.

58. Weingarten S, et al. Triage practice guideline for patients hospitalized with CHF: improving the effectiveness of the CCU. *Am J Med*. 1993;94:483–490.

59. Selker HP, et al. How do physicians adapt when the coronary care unit is full? A prospective multicenter study. *JAMA*. 1987;257:1181–1185.

60. Falk RP. Adverse reactions to medications on a coronary care unit. *Postgrad Med J*. 1979; 55:870–873.

61. Hackett TP, et al. The coronary-care unit: an appraisal of its psychologic hazards. *N Engl J Med*. 19;279:1365–1370.

62. Sykes DH, et al. Discharge from a coronary care unit: psychological factors. *J Psychosom Res*. 1989;33:477–488.

63. Bidell S, et al. Incidence and characteristics of preventable iatrogenic cardiac arrests. *JAMA*. 1991; 265:2815–2820.

64. Myers JD. Preventing iatrogenic complications. *N Engl J Med*. 1981;304:664–665.

65. Weingarten S, et al. Reducing lengths of stay in the coronary care unit with a practice guideline for patients with CHF: insights from a controlled clinical trial. *Med Care*. 1994;32:1232–1243.

66. Eddy DM. Practice policies: guidelines for methods. *JAMA*. 1990;263:1839–1841.

67. Guadagnoli E, et al. Outcomes research: hope for the future or the latest rage? *Inquiry*. 1994; 31:14–24.

68. Hays RD, et al. Psychometric evaluation and interpretation of health-related quality of life data. In: Schumaker S, Berzon R, eds. *The International Assessment of Health-Related Quality of Life: Theory, Translation, Measurement and Analysis*. Oxford, England: Rapid Communications; 1995:103–114.

69. Lembcke PA. Medical auditing by scientific methods: illustrated by major female pelvic surgery. *N Engl J Med*. 1956;162:646–655.

70. Owens D, et al. Development of outcome-based practice guidelines: a method for structuring problems and synthesizing evidence. *J Qual Improvement*. 1993;19:248–263.

71. Joint National Committee on Detection, Evaluation, and Treatment of High Blood Pressure. The fifth report of the Joint National Committee on detection, evaluation, and treatment of high blood pressure (JNC V). *Arch Intern Med*. 1993;153:154–183.

72. Diabetes Control and Complications Trial Research Group. The effect of intensive treatment of diabetes mellitus on the development and progression of long-term complications in insulin-dependent diabetes mellitus. *N Engl J Med*. 1993;329:977–986.

73. Reichard P, et al. The effect of long-term intensified insulin treatment on the development of microvascular complications of diabetes mellitus. *N Engl J Med*. 1993;329:304–309.

74. Wang PH, et al. Meta-analysis of effects of intensive blood-glucose control on late complications of type I diabetes. *Lancet*. 1993;341:1306–1309.

75. Zitter M. Disease management: a new approach to health care. *Med Interface*. August 1994: 70–76.

CHAPTER 4

The Role of Outcomes Management in Disease Management

Spencer Borden IV

Who is interested in outcomes management?

The measurement and management of outcomes have become key measures of process and results for all those engaged in disease management. The key users of outcomes information will be physicians, for both the management of medical delivery systems and the systematic analysis of clinical results of care. Beyond physicians, there is a broad range of users, including the numerous, diverse constituencies interested in outcomes measurement and management. Some potential users of outcomes measurements are

- patients
- providers
- provider groups
- hospitals
- managed-care organizations
- purchasing cooperatives
- employers/brokers
- accreditation agencies
- governmental agencies
- legal entities[1]

That a specific outcome of a disease management program can be measured does not mean that it needs to be measured. The key questions are: What *small number* of measures and outcomes are vitally important for the customer of the analytic study? What measures are sensitive measures of success for the project? What are measures of success for the enterprise as a whole? The answers to these questions are expected to be different because the chief executive officer will need different, enterprisewide measures of success than a physician executive, who has line management responsibility to manage the details of the disease management system.

In this regard, outcomes measurement is *the* critical evaluative tool for outcomes management. But the health care data analyst cannot design these critical measures in a vacuum. The outcomes measurement system requires critical thinking and input from the key customer: the physician manager of the disease management project.

A conceptual framework for outcomes measures can be constructed to provide to the critical audiences the opportunity to understand the diverse measures of outcomes and to gauge which measure might best serve their particular purpose. The model presented in Table 4–1 is for diabetes.

Outcomes measurements are part of broader quality improvement initiatives that include systems reengineering, process improvement, case management, and disease management. Some potential uses of outcomes measurements are

- clinical decision support
- tracking of patient progress
- assessing treatment effectiveness
- continuous quality improvement
- payment decisions

Table 4–1 A Framework of Outcome Measures for Diabetes

Outcome Domains	Outcome Measures
Process of care	Testing and screening
	Education
	Self-care
Clinical	Metabolic control
	Blood pressure control
	Weight control
	Morbidity and complications
Utilization/cost	Outpatient
	Inpatient
Patient satisfaction	Overall medical care
	Diabetes—specific treatment
Functional status/quality of life	General
	Dimension—specific
	Diabetes—specific

Courtesy of Value Health Services, Santa Monica, California.

- technology assessment
- marketing and sales
- licensing and accreditation
- program evaluation
- report cards
- provider credentialing
- provider profiling
- provider contracting[1]

Any such program must include the ability to measure the results of health care interventions in the following domains:

- medical management
- surgery
- physical rehabilitation
- drug therapy
- patient education
- behavior modification

Within and across each of these areas, there are focused and more specific uses of outcomes information, such as

- measuring the impact of care on a patient's health status and quality of life
- improving the decision-making process used by patients and clinicians
- evaluating the effectiveness of care and identifying opportunities for improvement[1]

Outcomes measurement is the key infrastructure of outcomes management. It requires the systematic collection and evaluation of health care data, intelligent data analysis, and production of measures of health care that can be tracked and trended for physician managers. Without such measurement no meaningful effort to influence clinical or financial outcomes can succeed.

COLLECTION AND EVALUATION OF HEALTH CARE DATA

Sources of Data

Health care data exist in many forms and at multiple locations of health care organizations. Physician executives must know where different types of health care data exist in their organization, the form and content of such data, and the uses for which such data could be valuable.

Existing sources of health care data need to be critically evaluated to determine if the desired measures of outcomes can be produced from them. Are these measures widely recognized and understood, or are they novel, requiring a new data and information infrastructure and new analytic processes to produce? If the existing data sources are inadequate, new sources of health care data must be found, or, more expensively, constructed from scratch. An effort should be launched to discover alternative, more easily produced measures of outcomes. In outcomes measurement and management, there is a constant tension between the desirability of newer, sophisticated measures of performance and the difficulty of routinely producing new measures.

In general, health care data exist in two forms: electronic (digitized in computers) and other (mainly paper).

Electronic Data Formats

To exchange electronic data between two sites and between two computers, sender and receiver must use and recognize a common format. Data formats must be defined using standard code conventions, definitions, and lengths of contained data elements.

Such data formats have been developed for claims data, the most prevalent type of electronic health care data. These claims data formats have been devised by payers and providers to assist in the payment transaction process. The use of claims data to measure health care performance or outcomes has only developed in the past 20 years. Such uses severely test the limits of the data content in claims data, originally designed only for payment purposes. However, the widespread availability of claims data in an electronic format has encouraged their use in health care measurement. Claims data are principally in three formats, depending on the site of care delivered and the type of service provided:

1. hospital inpatient and outpatient facility claims in UB-82 or UB-92 formats
2. professional claims in HCFA-1500 format
3. pharmaceutical claims using National Drug Codes (NDCs)

Electronic data formats have also been developed for function-specific systems, such as laboratory reporting systems within hospitals, and for integrated delivery systems (ie, electronic data interchanges [EDIs]).

Hospital Claims Data. The UB-82 and UB-92 (Uniform Billing, 1982 and 1992) formats were devised by the Health Care Financing Administration (HCFA) for submission of hospital bills to Medicare. Hospitals now submit their facility claims to all payers using these formats. The hospital's billing systems are capable of producing electronic tapes of all hospital charges for external collection and analysis by payers, state regulatory agencies, state data agencies, review organizations, health care researchers, and consultants.

The key data fields available on UB-82 and UB-92 formats include:

- the name, age, gender, and zip code of the patient
- codes identifying the attending physician and operating surgeon
- the principal diagnosis and up to four secondary diagnoses (in codes using the International Classification of Disease System, 9th or 10th version [ICD-9 or ICD-10])
- the procedures the patient underwent (in codes using the Common Procedural Terminology Codes, version 4 [CPT-4])
- raw measures of patient outcome (discharged alive, discharged to nursing home, or died)
- billed charges and length of stay
- payer of record

Radiology, laboratory, pharmaceutical, and nursing (ancillary) charges are usually compiled in aggregate categories using nonstandard definitions. These are less easily available for analysis and comparison.

These claims records can be catalogued into diagnosis-related groups (DRGs) using the principal and secondary diagnoses, the patient's age, and complications, including death. DRGs were originally developed at Yale as a research method to examine patterns of hospital resource utilization. They were later adopted by the state of New Jersey and then by HCFA. They are now the method used for payment for Medicare patients and by payers in selected states.

DRGs are an excellent example of the creation of *derivative files:* aggregation of raw claims data into meaningful groupings that provide an excellent opportunity for further analysis and comparison (and even payment). In large part, the sophistication in the use of claims data in health care measurement and comparison has developed in parallel with the development of sophisticated derivative claims data files, which use expert systems to create higher levels of information than contained in large amounts of raw claims data. Other examples of derivative files include alternative diagnostic groupings of patients, such as the *all-patient refined diagnosis-related groups* (APR-DRGs), the groupings of patients by disease-specific severity and comorbidity levels, and the creation of episodes of illness, which define time periods during which the diagnosis and treatment of a patient's disease typically occurs. The great advantages in the use of derivative files are the compression of data by the derivative files, the intelligence used in their creation, and the comparability of data across delivery sites if the groupers are correctly applied to accurate data.

Professional Claims Data. Physicians and their practice groups submit professional claims to payers in the HCFA-1500 format. Although some claims are still submitted on paper, most are submitted in electronic format by tape-to-tape transfer. The key data elements in HCFA-1500 claims are

- the identity of the patient
- the identity of the physician (typically the tax identification number, or TIN, of the physician or the practice group)
- the services provided in CPT-4 codes
- the diagnosis in ICD-9 codes
- the charge for the services
- the date of service

Two major difficulties exist in professional claims data. One physician may have multiple TINs if he or she practices in multiple locations and bills payers through the TIN of different practice organizations. Some physician practices bill all services for all their physicians using the TIN of the practice entity, effectively lumping all individual physician performance together in an aggregate measure that averages out individual practitioners' performance. A recent study of death and complication rates of Medicare patients undergoing angioplasty procedures performed by high- and low-volume cardiologists showed 2.2% greater death and complications in low-volume cardiologists. This study was made possible only by Medicare's requirement that all doctors submit their individual identification numbers with their bills.[2] The diagnosis is frequently omitted from professional claims, hindering analysts from determining the clinical rationale for the service being billed.

Professional claims data are the most useful, widely available source of data on how physicians actually practice and what resources are used in their decisions on diagnosis, treatment, and monitoring of patients' conditions. In more evolved and sophisticated forms of managed care, these information resources are very necessary but are increasingly unavailable. In staff-model HMOs, physicians are typically on yearly salaries and have no need to submit professional claims. Similarly, under capitation arrangements, physicians are paid with a per-member per-month (PMPM) stipend, without regard to how much care, if any, the member actually receives. In delivery systems with well-developed capitation payment methods, the lack of actual cost and utilization data on physician practice patterns can prevent any analysis and management of the variations and patterns of professional practice. In such systems, physicians may be required to submit dummy claims data ("encounter forms"). But in the absence of any financial consequence for noncompliance, many physicians ignore this obligation.

Pharmaceutical Claims Data. Pharmaceutical claims are submitted for those patients covered by a pharmacy benefit plan, usually as a health benefit of full-time employment. Insurance carriers or pharmacy benefit management (PBM) companies process and pay the claims. Typically, over-the-counter medications are not included in the pharmacy plan and are paid out of pocket by the patient. This utilization is not reflected in pharmaceutical claims data.

Medications in pharmacy claims are coded by National Drug Codes (NDCs), a broad coding system for classes of medications. Individual or brand-specific medications may not be identifiable in pharmacy claims data sets. Pharmacy claims data do not confirm compliance of the patient in taking all the medications as prescribed; they only confirm the purchase of the medication.

Pharmaceutical claims data, particularly in PBMs, are not correlated with other medical claims data on the same patient. They are separately processed and archived and have different patient identifiers, making the linkage of claims data for the same patient very difficult.

Data from Function-Specific Systems. In delivery systems with good computerization of information, such as hospitals, function-specific computerized information may be available for capture and analysis. Laboratory reporting systems can provide timely outputs of laboratory values directly to the patient's nurses on the hospital floor and to the medical record. Such reports may include normal expected values and trended laboratory results over the patient's hospital stay. Similarly, radiology information systems can schedule examinations, provide algorithms for exam sequencing, and allow the radiologist's report to be electronically sent to the patient's chart or to the office of the referring physician. Similar systems exist for physician order entry, pharmacy services, and adverse event reporting.

The electronic outputs of such data systems need to be integrated with data from other sources and correctly mapped by patient identifier to allow valid consolidation of clinical and utilization data.

Electronic Data Interchange Transaction Data. Electronic data interchanges (EDIs) are electronic systems connecting providers, hospitals, payers, employers, and third-party administrators (TPAs) to capture and process transactions of health care services provided for employed patients. Such systems are not commonly in place but are seen as the future data infrastructure of integrated delivery systems. Covered patients are provided with magnetic or "smart" (containing a computer chip) cards confirming their identity, their employer, the type of benefit plan covering them, and the TPA processing their claims. At every locus of care, the patient's card is swiped through an electronic card reader that contains the site of care, the type of service, the provider, and the charge. These data may pass to the employer for verification of coverage, to the TPA for repricing and payment under terms of the patient's benefit plan, and to the provider's account for electronic fund transfer, typically within 24 hours. Comprehensive transaction data are collected in a central data file.

EDI systems have multiple advantages over conventional systems. They capture all transactions, including

- over-the-counter medications
- claims for services that may not be paid because services are outside the scope of the plan and are thus not covered
- claims for which the deductible or copay limits may not have been met
- claims that properly fall within auto liability or workers' compensation (subrogation)
- claims denied because of alternative benefit coverage (coordination of benefits)
- claims from noncontracted providers in a managed-care plan

A complete, accurate, and detailed patient utilization and cost profile can be constructed and maintained by EDI systems. When operating in conjunction with smart cards containing patients' diagnoses, lab and radiology results, medications, allergies, a synopsis of clinical data, and dates of next scheduled visits, EDI systems promise to capture rich clinical data to enhance utilization and cost profiles.

Nonelectronic Data Formats

Hospital Medical Record Data. Hospital medical records are widely considered to be the gold standard of clinical information, leading to sophistication in the measurement of clinical outcomes. The hospital medical record collects comprehensive information from multiple sources, including

- medical history
- physical exam
- physicians' progress notes
- nursing notes
- operative notes
- pharmacy, laboratory, and radiology results

All the above are contained in standard locations in the patient's hospital record. Such data are reviewed by multiple caregivers and are considered to be very accurate. Detailed clinical data have been widely required in the appropriate use of explicit outcome methods.[3] The recent emphasis on careful documentation of the patient's status has only served to improve the quality of hospital record information.

However, the use of hospital medical record data to measure clinical outcomes has many obstacles. By definition, hospital records cover only inpatient admissions, making measurement across inpatient and outpatient delivery sites very difficult. Hospital records are largely in paper, not electronic, formats. Thus, hospital medical record information needs to be manually abstracted to be captured for measurement. This process is labor intensive and expensive. To perform hospital abstracting, the regional differences in medical nomenclature need to be addressed by the use of a glossary to translate equivalent terms. The very profusion of data in the hospital medical record requires the careful selection of the key data elements to be used in measurement of clinical outcomes. Two types of clinical markers have been developed to measure patient severity of illness from hospital medical records:

1. generic, non–disease-specific severity measures
2. disease-specific measures, such as for coronary artery bypass surgery[4]

The former are criticized because they are insensitive to unusual presentations of particular diseases and the latter because the same severity measure cannot be used to compare severity levels across diseases. No nationally recognized standard of severity measurement exists.

The electronic medical record, although desirable from many perspectives, is not yet in widespread use. Portions of the hospital medical record lend themselves to electronic formats and transmission. Pharmacy, laboratory, and radiology information and reporting systems can be captured on patient records at computers in multiple sites of care delivery in the hospital. Two additional problems complicate the widespread use of the electronic medical record. First, a universal patient identifier code permitting multiple organizations to exchange patient-specific information into a single electronic record has not been developed and accepted. Second, confidentiality of patient information has been a difficult issue for health care information systems. Patient confidentiality can be protected by controlling access to patient-specific information on a need-to-know basis. From the perspective of health care data analysts, patient names can be coded for anonymity. Groups of patients in a specific category are necessary for statistical measures of performance. Isolated patients in a specific disease category could be identified, but these patients are anecdotes of delivery care and cannot be statistically summarized.

Outpatient Medical Record Data. Outpatient medical records have suffered from multiple levels of inconsistency. Most are collected in paper format and have the same problems as paper medical records of hospital admissions. Outpatient records are frequently handwritten and difficult to read and may lack the comprehensive collection of data from outside ancillary testing and procedures. They may be poorly available to other office locales or for emergencies and may be kept in nonstandardized formats. Patients may be identified by name, social security number, or relationships in families (often used for children). Such idiosyncracies prevent easy collection of patient data across different sites of health care delivery.

There have been several attempts to create a standard outpatient medical record in electronic format. These endeavors have struggled with the degree of accuracy and comprehensiveness required of the record and with data fields that must be filled in by the provider. There is also the difficulty of capturing free text into the record. Standardization of patient description, diagnosis, and therapeutic plans may constrain individual commentary. Information system design problems arise in the capture of patient information from ancillary sources, from other practice locations, and from specialist referrals. The problems of outpatient medical records must be addressed and solved during the further consolidation of health care delivery organizations and the development of integrated delivery systems.

Patient Self-Reports of Status (SF-36). Over the past decade, the value of patient-supplied data has been explored. Three broad categories of patient-generated data exist: the patient's health status, the quality of life or well-being of the patient, and patient satisfaction survey results. These data are obtainable only from direct patient responses to focused questionnaires and surveys.

Patients have been surveyed for satisfaction with health care delivery processes (access, waiting time, completeness and clarity of explanation by the physician, etc) and with the service component of care delivery. Although often asked of patients, reports of satisfaction with the technical aspects of care are unreliable and frequently colored by the satisfaction with health care service.

Patient functional status has proven to be highly informative and to correlate well with objective measures of clinical outcomes. Through the use of a publicly available survey instrument, the Short Form 36 questionnaire (SF-36), patient responses to 36 standard questions have been assessed.[5] The functional status of individual patients or cohorts of patients can be tracked, trended, and compared to national samples of similar responses. The SF-36 instrument has opened a new avenue of exploration of patient-perceived results of care. Self-reported outcomes of care can be used to define expected functional results of care and to search for prevalence of complications, incomplete recovery or rehabilitation from surgery, or comorbid factors that might adversely affect the patient's functional status.

The SF-36 must be administered to patients and the results collected and tabulated. The data are best used when correlated with other measures of health care performance; this means that common patient identifiers are required to compile the information from multiple sources. The use of touch-screen computer technologies may facilitate the collection and tabulation of SF-36 patient data and promote their integration into systematic measures of health care performance.

As would be expected with any new measure of clinical outcome, a recent study using the SF-36 on smaller select patient cohorts, namely, the elderly and the poor and chronically ill, demonstrated worse physical health outcomes among health maintenance organization (HMO) patients than among fee-for-service (FFS) system patients.[6]

Patient functional status may also be measured by specific disease category. The standard SF-36 questions may be augmented by disease-specific questions to probe the results of care for patients with a common disease condition. There are multiple initiatives across the United States to use and standardize these disease-specific approaches. The Health Outcomes Institute (formerly of Interstudy and now part of Stratis Health, Inc., in Minnesota) has developed the TyPE (Technology of Patient Experience) system to elicit disease-specific functional status for selected diseases. These data have been combined with medical record data and trended over years of observation. The use of such information allows different cohorts of patients with a disease in common to be compared and evaluated against a national sample of similar patients. Regional variations in care or best practices leading to superior functional outcomes could be discovered in such comparisons.

Issues of Data Integrity and Comparability

Isolated Data Sets with No Common Identifier

Most health care data sets have been designed and created to accomplish one specific purpose. A cancer registry collects information on only those patients who have a form of cancer. Pharmaceutical claims data are designed to pay for a purchase transaction of a medication. A radiology scheduling system is designed to track and speed the flow of patients through a busy radiology department. Data are captured and stored in a form and in a distribution system that supports their central purpose. In large measure, health care data systems were not designed to integrate with other data systems, so the process of linking independent data systems to accomplish a new, derivative application is difficult.

A common identifier, or data element, is required to link separate data systems. The common identifier must be accurately recorded in each of the linked systems; otherwise, a false linkage of unrelated data is created. The common identifier must be an important unit of measurement for the purposes of the analysis. The creation of linked data sets of patient care delivery using the hospital identifier as the common data element might be helpful to the hospital's medical director or financial officer but would be of little value to a researcher examining the longitudinal course of a patient's treatment of a particular disease.

The most common approach to linking health care data sets is to use a common patient identifier from different databases. This approach is highly desirable, as patients can be aggregated by disease, severity level, location of care, use of a particular technology, or clinical outcome to yield valuable information.

In practice, most databases use different, unique patient codes to identify individual patients. Thus, the data integration challenge focuses on how an individual patient can be properly identified in different data sets. There is no widely used, nationally recognized, unique, coded patient identifier in existence. Therefore, secondary patient characteristics are often used in these mapping exercises. Social Security Administration number (SSAN) codes are helpful but are not one of a kind and are not applicable to children under 1 year old. (Children over 1 year are required to have social security numbers for their parent's tax returns). Date of birth is often used but does not discriminate between twin siblings born on the same date. Mother's first name or maiden name can help, but names and nicknames can change. ZIP code of residence location is subject to change when a family moves and is not useful in cases of homeless people. Using the best mapping strategies to combine different patient identifiers for the same patient between different databases yields a match rate on the order of 70%. Optimists might claim that most of the patient sample was preserved. Pessimists would regard the loss of 30% of the sample size as unacceptable.

Data Accuracy and Completeness

The fact that data exist in a database somewhere in the organization does not mean that they are usable. By itself, primary data collection is a tedious and repetitive process. If collected by human beings in an interactive process, the pressures of time and work flows may cause shortcuts to be taken, such as

- failure to fill necessary data fields (incompleteness)
- insertion of wrong codes for patient, payer, procedure, or diagnostic group (inaccuracy)
- application of codes that are mutually inconsistent between gender of the patient and diagnosis or procedure (incompatibility)
- filling required data fields with a series of zeros or nines

These errors, individually and collectively, degrade the value of a set of data to be meaningfully analyzed.

Organizations that routinely process health care data in the production of analyses or reports have developed software programs to screen the accuracy and completeness of databases to be analyzed. These expert systems measure the location and prevalence of incompleteness, inaccuracy, or incompatibility in the database considered for analysis. Depending on the results of such expert data quality analysis, one of three options may be selected. If the data quality is acceptable (to both the analyst and customer of the analysis), the analysis may proceed. If the data quality is substandard, can the data be corrected or augmented with accurate, new data sources? If so, the databases should be enhanced and data quality measured again. If not, the lack of satisfactory data may preclude the analysis.

Issues of Data Storage and Retrieval

If data are considered a valuable asset, storing data for reuse should be a priority. To some, storing data in electronic formats is a simple challenge to access enough computer memory to handle the volume of data to be stored. Compression codes can collapse many repetitive sequences of electronic data by using secondary codes to represent far longer sequences of data bits, resulting in 30% to 50% reductions in required memory space. The evolution of storage technology has allowed vast improvements in memory capacity, together with a dramatic reduction in cost. In such memory systems, data retrieval is a process to download large quantities of raw data to smaller computers for refinement and analysis.

The use of derivative files of data has complicated the issues of data storage and retrieval. Using complicated algorithms, derivative files assemble data elements into groups of data that contain secondary characteristics and enhance the ability to do comparisons within and between databases. Examples of derivative files are familiar to many:

- diagnosis-related groups (DRGs)
- major diagnostic categories (MDCs)
- groupers of severity and comorbidity
- ambulatory care groups (ACGs)
- ICD-9 codes
- CPT-4 codes

These derivative files are continuously evolving conventions on how to aggregate data to create groups of data containing higher levels of information.

Storing data containing derivative files imposes new burdens upon the organization. First, the version of the grouper must be captured and maintained in the documentation of the stored data so that analysts in the future will understand the conventions used in the creation of the stored derivative files. Second, the raw data (at the claim-line level) must be kept, usually in archival or inactive storage. These raw data may need to be accessed in studies using both current and historical, stored data.

Analyses of performance over time (trend reports) may cross the time horizons in which an early version of a data grouper is replaced by a later version. Failure to recognize that a grouper has changed during the study period will lead to erroneous results because the derivative files being compared are not identical. So the analyst must access the historical data; regroup the historical, raw data, using the current version of the grouper; and perform the trend analysis. This regrouping process requires time and money to access the data, recalculate the derivative files, perform the trend analysis, and store the updated files. If trend reporting is infrequent, such regroupings may be performed on an as-needed basis. However, if trend reporting is routine and involves most of a stored claims database, yearly regroupings of the entire historical database, using the most recent grouper version, may be more cost-effective than "as-needed" regrouping efforts.

Issues of Confidentiality

Patients have a right to have their information kept confidential, but measurement of health care performance requires the use of patient information. To the casual observer, this tug-of-war is not resolvable, so patient files should be kept under lock and key. The apparent confidentiality problem can be solved, however, once the desired uses of the data and the functions of those people with legitimate access to the data files are understood.

A key consideration here is the unit of analysis under consideration. If an analysis is investigating the cost and utilization profile of patients with a particular disease, each patient under active medical management will have a cost and utilization profile and will contribute one patient's experience (observation) to the analysis. Every hospitalized patient will have a length of stay expressed in days. If exploratory surgery of the abdomen is the unit of analysis, a large population will be needed to collect enough surgical experience to analyze. Most patients will provide no observations to this surgical analysis. If very rare events are the unit of analysis, such as medical services leading to medical liability lawsuits, a very large population will be required to assemble enough observations to be credible.

For statistical analysis, any single patient is an experience of one. One patient's experience is an anecdote: informative but not conclusive. Aggregations of patients are required for statistical analysis. Patient groups of fewer than 30 persons have high levels of statistical uncertainty (standard deviations). To measure differences in health care outcomes that may differ by 10%, patient groups of 100 individuals or more may be needed. To measure outcomes that may differ by as little as 1%, thousands of patients are needed. Patients in these analyses are best used in aggregated forms, such as diagnostic groups. In such analyses, once the critical mass of patients is achieved, the next issue is the comparability of patients. This is usually addressed through the use of derivative files of patient groupings. Thus, for both the health care data analyst and the user of the analytical report, the adequacy of patient volumes and the acceptability of the resulting uncertainty, given the magnitude of the difference sought, must be understood and accepted.

Patients with rare or exotic medical conditions rarely exist in sufficient numbers to allow statistical analysis of their experience and are avoided by skilled health care analysts. However, even with a coded patient identifier, the experience of a single such patient must not be publicly released, since the very rarity of his or her condition may allow his or her identity to be deduced.

Patient-specific data are needed at almost all levels of health care data analysis. Patients are the most valuable unit of analysis. Therefore, patient-level data must be sought and stored. Patients are identified by name in text files and by coded identifier in most electronic claims formats. Unplanned public release of patient-specific data in coded form is regrettable but will not jeopardize patient confidentiality if the key containing the text name equivalents of the coded identifiers is not released as well. Such text files of patient names and the key to the coded identifiers should be securely stored and accessible only to those with need-to-know security clearance to examine the files.

The system design issues with need-to-know security clearances are beyond the scope of this discussion. But the issue of need-to-know clearances is of paramount importance in the design and function of outcomes analysis of disease management initiatives. If addressed proactively and processed correctly, need-to-know security clearances will minimize the possibility of breach of patient confidentiality and ensure that skilled analysts and physician managers have appropriate access to the information that they require.

ANALYSIS OF HEALTH CARE DATA

Purpose

Health care data analysis is a skilled manipulation of collected data to explore variances and provide measures of performance. However, that definition misses the central, practical point of doing health care data analysis. What is the central purpose of the analysis? Exactly what is being explored? How will the outputs of the analysis be read and used? How certain must the result be? What difference will the analysis make in the practical delivery of health care services to the covered population? The answers to these questions must be known to the skilled health care analyst because they determine the approach to query the data, the degree of uncertainty that is acceptable, the formats of the resulting analysis, and the customers of the analytic results.

Tactics

Given the answers to the above questions, the skilled health data analyst will choose the appropriate collection of patients to examine and the criteria for their inclusion in the study. Are the selected measures of performance accurate and valid indices of the desired performance? Dividing the yearly number of outpatient visits to a hospital by the square footage of its parking lots may yield a useful index for a traffic control officer but little relevant information to the physician executive. Is the patient population large enough to answer the relevant performance measures at the required level of certainty? Is the demographic mix of patients appropriate for the type of performance measure sought by the analyst? Are the sources of data comprehensive enough to support the breadth of performance measures to be applied?

The skill sets required of the sophisticated health care data analyst are numerous:

- familiarity with the types of input data feeds, their construction, and their level of accuracy
- in-depth knowledge of applied statistics and processes of data manipulation
- the types and uses of derivative databases
- understanding of the health care delivery system and its relational components
- the ability to communicate the analytical results in verbal, tabular, graphical, and numerical formats

Study Period

The time period of the analysis is a critical dimension. Large groups of patients with acute, short-term illnesses could be profiled with one or two quarters of a year's data experience, but rare illnesses with a chronic course of disease progression would require a larger patient base over a far longer period of observation. Longer retrospective data analyses trade more accuracy in precision of the analysis against greater irrelevancy of the measures as the time period of the analysis recedes from the present. The managerial use of the data analyses will determine the value of precision versus the timeliness of the analysis.

Patient Characteristics

The level of sophistication of the analysis will determine the appropriateness of the use of derivative files of patient characteristics. Is patient grouping by DRGs, clusters of ICD-9 codes (sometimes called "disease types" or "conditions"), or location of provision of services the best method of lumping together the results of patient experience? As the definition of patient grouping is restricted, the population available for study becomes smaller, and the time required to collect enough patients to satisfy criteria for statistical certainty of the results expands.

Even within diagnostic clusters of patients, patient characteristics of severity of illness and the presence of comorbid conditions will raise questions of the comparability of patient populations. Should these patient characteristics be measured and included in the analysis? If so, are these measures code based, available using algorithms to sort claims data, or medical record based, using the results of medical history, physical examination, laboratory findings, and radiological and clinical pathology results? If medical record–based measures of severity are required, are the necessary measures disease-specific markers of patient severity or generic measures of severity that apply across different disease conditions? Both publicly available and proprietary systems of severity and comorbidity measures are available. Most disease management organizations do not have the time or expertise to develop these measures on their own, so outside sources of severity and comorbidity are used for analyses requiring these adjustments.

Oversampling of High-Risk Populations

In large populations with relatively healthy people, the proportion of patients who are in high-risk categories or who sustain unfavorable outcomes may be very small. If a sampling approach is taken to measure outcomes in such a population, the overwhelming number of healthy patients may overpower the small number of unfavorable outcomes, yielding a result with no statistical significance. A preferred approach is to oversample the high-risk patients, compared to the low-risk population. With this strategy, small proportions of unfavorable results will not be lost but will be sensitively measured. Clearly, the oversampling strategy can only be extended to include the entire population of high-risk patients. It is not applicable when the entire population is included and those results are measured.

Episodes of Care

Episodes of care are periods of time during which the diagnostic process and therapeutic course of a disease are completed. Originally used in the RAND Health Insurance Experiment in the 1980s, episodes of care have been widely accepted and are now the preferred method of collapsing a diversity of health care services together to profile the pattern of diagnosis and treatment of a particular disease. The episode-of-care methodology is best used with claims data, since data are collected from multiple sites of care, using multiple types of services from multiple providers of care. Medical record data are difficult to collapse across inpatient and outpatient delivery locations.

The definition of the appropriate length of time for an episode of care for a particular disease is controversial. Episodes that are short may capture only those services relevant to the disease under analysis. However, they risk losing those later services, referable to the index disease, that fall outside the episode window of analysis, causing false-negative conclusions. Conversely, episodes that tend to be longer capture all the relevant services for a disease condition but risk including unrelated services within the profile of disease diagnosis and treatment, causing false-positive conclusions.

Other episode definitions have been advocated. Variable-length episodes of care have been defined as those periods of time under which patients are under active medical management. The episode is closed only when a patient receives no medical services for a defined period. The advantage of variable-length episodes of care is that they are patient specific, reflecting individual patients' response to treatment. The disadvantage is that the nonstandard length of the episode confounds the comparison of different patients treated by different physicians.

Norms or Standards

The use of norms or averages is desirable for most studies. More insight can be gained by comparing the results of the analysis to a standard of some sort. But what is the "right" standard to use? For those analyses for which there is no relevant external measure with which to compare, the results can only be compared within the variances of the study population. The measured performance can be said to be at, above, or below the "community" average. These results may have little meaningful impact on those practitioners near the middle of the bell-shaped curve but will be informative to those at the high or low ends of the distribution. For purposes of physician education and quality improvement, local or network-based measures of performance are the most meaningful. Most physicians consider their local colleagues as peers and prefer to be compared to them. External measures of performance can be derived from statewide, regional, or national data sources, but most physicians will consider the standards of performance in delivery systems remote from their community to be so different from those of their own community as to be irrelevant for comparison purposes.

Benchmarks or Best Practices

To be compared to levels of average performance is not very challenging. By definition, half the delivery units under analysis will be above the average. The likely response to the news of above-average performance is to compliment the measurement system on the accuracy of the results and to engage in self-congratulation. A better response would be to challenge the delivery unit to emulate the performance of the best-in-class delivery units.

What are the results that might be considered benchmark or best in class? The delivery system with the very best results is at the apex of performance but, as a standard, would be considered unattainable by most delivery units, especially by those below the mean. What levels of performance are superior, considered benchmark, but still attainable by other delivery units?

Two standard deviations from the mean in a favorable direction might be considered benchmark performance. It is highly regarded and statistically different from the average performance. But in random distribution of results, this level would include only 5% of all units measured and might be seen as unattainable by the other 95% of the measured units.

Arbitrary levels of benchmark performance are more easily defined and accepted. Performance at the 75th or 80th percentile is considered admirable, includes 20% to 25% of all units above the benchmark threshold, and is considered "within reach" by delivery systems with lower performance levels. The creation of such benchmark thresholds is no problem for the experienced health care data analyst.

Variation from the Mean

Another analytic consideration is the degree of variability of performance within a measured group. If the accepted standard is the average performance for a group of patients, variation in performance will be described in terms of variation from the mean. In statistical terms, such variations can be described in measurements of standard deviations from the mean. *Statistical significance* is defined as variations measured at greater than two standard deviations from the mean. In human terms, variation in performance will be expressed in clinical outcomes markedly different from the average, in either a favorable or an unfavorable direction.

There are three interpretative issues with measures of variability to be addressed:

1. Statistical significance of variation from the mean may not be required if physician managers are going to use the results to target corrective measures. Smart physician executives can use trends of performance and performance results that are diverging from the expected as indicators to intervene in the health care delivery process; statistical certainty of difference from the average is not required.
2. The use of standard deviations implies that the performance results are distributed randomly and that the past year's results will not influence the degree of variance or distribution of this year's results. These hypotheses are not widely acknowledged, nor are they widely accepted for health care delivery systems.
3. The widespread variations in performance results may imply that the underlying systems are not in control, being subject to both the "normal" variation in outcomes and the variability caused by extraordinary causes. If this is true, these factors would indicate that any corrective actions taken by management will have no remedial effect but will serve only to increase the observed variability in performance.

PRODUCTION OF MEASURES

Process Measures

Process measures in health care delivery are those service steps that are taken in the prevention, diagnosis, and treatment of disease conditions. Clearly, process steps that are generated routinely are the easiest to capture and measure. Process steps in the delivery of health care delivery services are intended to improve the condition of the patient and to favorably affect the consequences of disease. But the linkage of discrete process steps with direct improvement in patient outcomes is missing for almost all types of process steps. One exception is childhood immunization against infectious disease. Immunization of children increases resistance to specific diseases and, in the aggregate, prevents their occurrence. For a specific child, immunization is expected to improve clinical resistance to infectious disease, but the specific benefit of improved outcomes for that child will not be proven for decades. There is also the risk of adverse results from the immunization process itself.

Financial Measures of Process: Costs and Its Variations

Since most process steps in service delivery to patients trigger a financial cost that has to be processed and paid, financial measurement of health care delivery processes is well developed and understood. The advantage of financial measures of process is that all process steps can be measured with a common yardstick: dollars. At this point, the simplicity ends.

A cost of a health care service could be considered the cost of production of that service, a sum of the direct and indirect costs of its completion. This is the cost to the organization providing the service. Provider organizations may know their costs in the aggregate (total expenses) or by line of service (e.g., radiology department in a hospital) but not at the level of an individual service (e.g., a single chest X-ray examination).

A price is the fee that the delivery organization submits to a payer after provision of a health care service (e.g., a charge for a completed chest X-ray). It is a sticker price. The actual paid amount may be very different from the sticker price. Sticker prices are often discounted by contractual discounts between the provider and the payer, or they may be replaced by a fee schedule mutually agreed upon by both parties in advance. The paid amount may be differently shared between the payer and the patient, depending on the terms of the benefit plan, the coordination of benefits between two employers, the subrogation of auto-related claims, the different coverage for services in and outside a managed-care network, or the application of copays, deductibles, or lifetime maximum allowables. Clearly, the exact definition of paid amounts is critical in health care analysis.

Utilization and Its Variants

Beginning with fee for service, each delivered service generates its own claim, to be submitted for payment. In capitated systems, such service-based claims are not necessary and are frequently not collected. For capitated delivery systems, encounter data are the equivalent to a health care claim, requiring similar data elements, with either $0 or $1 on the encounter form. The capture of comprehensive encounter data is a problem for many capitated managed care firms and their providers, whose income is not affected by the submission or lack of submission of encounter data.

Utilization data capture the use by patients of a similar type of service: examples are hospital admissions, visits to emergency departments, and physician office visits. The advantages of utilization data are that they are routinely collected, are readily understood by people familiar with delivery systems, and reflect actual units of work provided to patients. Within types of utilization, different levels of service or intensity are captured by CPT-4 codes (in physician office visits), days in routine care or intensive care (for hospital admissions), or CPT-4 codes of multiple procedures in a surgical service.

Utilization may relate to the locus of care (inpatient, outpatient, day surgery, etc) or to a specific type of service (chest X-rays, pharmaceutical prescriptions, laboratory tests, etc). One concern in health data analysis is the accuracy and comparability of coding of types of services rendered that, if inaccurate, would render the results highly suspect. The use of utilization data in health care analysis will depend on the appropriate use of patient stratification to adjust for patient-related factors of severity and comorbidity. The use of utilization data is rate based, requiring a denominator for the fraction to create ratios of use of a service per hospital admission or per total dollars spent. The use of a total population (both claimants and nonclaimants) as the denominator will yield data expressed as per-member per-month (PMPM) utilization figures (hospital admission per 1000 members, emergency department visits per 1000 members, etc). By definition, utilization data reflect units of work that were provided for patient care, as opposed to what should have been provided for that patient's care (a measure of appropriateness of service).

Pharmaceutical Profiles and Utilization

Claims for pharmaceutical prescriptions represent a parallel system of transactions from other medical and surgical claims. Drug claims for filled prescriptions are submitted to pharmacy claims processors or, more commonly, to pharmacy benefit management companies, rather than to traditional carriers and TPAs. As a consequence, the ability of pharmaceutical utilization data to enrich the information from medical and surgical claims data has not been widely appreciated. As previously mentioned, the issue of patient identification on the two data sets can be solved either by using a common patient code or by mapping patients by distinctive characteristics.

The use of pharmaceuticals in the management of disease can map very accurately the practice patterns of individual physicians, both in the frequency of pharmaceutical use in patients with specific diseases (incidence of use) and in the distribution of pharmaceuticals used for a disease condition (distribution of use). Mapping the types of pharmaceuticals used in the treatment of the disease condition by severity level can show types of pharmaceutical usage that are clearly not indicated (inappropriate) or are only marginally indicated.

Combining pharmaceutical claim information with medical claim diagnostic codes can validate the coded diagnosis. An example is the use of an oral hypoglycemic agent in a patient with a coded diagnosis of diabetes. Even better, the analysis of pharmaceutical usage can segment patients into meaningful prognostic categories. Another example is the use of insulin to identify patients with type I (insulin-dependent) diabetes, who are very different in treatment and prognosis from type II (non–insulin-dependent) diabetic patients.

Compliance with Screening Tests and Treatment Plans

The best medical plan to treat an illness will be jeopardized if the patient, for any reason, fails to comply with the instructions to complete the treatment plan. Compliance rates are a valid measure of process in patient care. Examples include compliance with timing and dosage of medications to be taken, compliance with follow-up visits with physicians or other health professionals, and completion of routine screening tests, such as yearly physical examinations.

Disease-Specific Process Measures

For many disease conditions, key measures of process have been widely considered to represent a minimal level of acceptable service, usually shown by scientific studies as leading to favorable outcomes. Pap smears, mammography screening, glycosylated hemoglobin levels, yearly measures of blood pressure, and triglyceride and cholesterol tests are examples of disease-specific measures of compliance with expectations that patients complete their scheduled services to monitor their diseases. The great advantage of these measures of process is that every qualified patient should have one of these process steps in the management of his or her disease within the defined time period, generating many points of observation for analysis. Compliance measures have an ideal value, namely, 100%, in their construction. The actual compliance rates usually fall far short of 100%. This gap, the opportunity potential for improvement, can be exactly quantified and specified for multiple levels in the delivery system (the managed care health plan as a whole, a group of physicians by geography or practice group, or at the level of the individual physician). The opportunity for process improvement and, implicitly, outcome improvement is easily seen. For these reasons, such measures have served as the mainstay of quality measures in the Health Plan Employer Data and Information Set (HEDIS) system of evaluation of managed care plans.

Patient Satisfaction

With the advent of patient-centered care and consideration of the patient as the customer of health care, surveys of patients' expectations, perceptions of care delivered, and satisfaction with rendered care are more often being undertaken by provider organizations. The results of such surveys are used in accreditation and in the marketing of a delivery system.

There has been a general skepticism concerning the results of the accuracy and comparability of such survey information from patients, due to its very subjective nature and the fact that patient responses are largely shaped by the comparison of patients' experience with their expectations of service. But, enough patient survey experience has been gained to show that survey results are consistent; show variances among providers, provider groups, and health care plans; and reflect overall patient experience with delivery systems. To that extent, survey results are very useful in measuring patients' response to their health care delivery and to the quality of service rendered to them.

For organizations whose focus is on service to customers, patient satisfaction survey results are critical in identifying opportunities to improve levels of customer service, to trend comparative performance over time, and to use in marketing and advertising new business from employers and patients.

Patient survey results may be affected by the wording of the questions asked, the timing of the questionnaire relative to the services in question (the sooner the better), and the technology of soliciting patient's responses (computer screen, telephone, letters to patient's homes, etc). The comparability of patient responses across different delivery systems and using different survey technology is an active area of investigation.

Provider Satisfaction

Patients are not the only interested participants in the health care delivery process. Physicians, other health care professionals, and office staff are good observers of the processes of care delivery. They may be considered internal customers of the delivery system. Processes of care that make their work more difficult or less fulfilling will elicit negative responses on surveys of providers.

Patient Knowledge

Some patients may have little or no knowledge of their disease condition, especially if the onset has been recent. Other patients with chronic illnesses may acquire detailed knowledge of their condition, perhaps due to their own inquisitive nature, a family history of the disease, or a support group formed by other patients with the disease, not to mention access to "chat rooms" on the Internet.

From a medical management perspective, greater patient knowledge is highly desirable for many reasons. Patients who understand the manifestations of their disease can be highly alert to subtle changes in their medical condition and their response to new therapies. They can be on watch for complications of therapeutic procedures or medications. Compliance with medication schedules, tests, procedures, and office visits is greater among knowledgeable patients. Also, greater patient disease knowledge can allow greater patient self-care and flexibility in the management of the disease, leading to lower costs of professional treatments. Clinical follow-up of highly knowledgeable patients can be performed over the telephone.

Measures of patients' knowledge of their disease condition before the intervention of a disease management program will show the relative skill sets of the patient population being considered for the intervention. Such measures can target those patient cohorts or individual patients who would most benefit from disease-specific education in the natural history of the disease and its treatment. For disease-specific management programs, initial measures of patient knowledge of disease will serve as the baseline from which gains in knowledge of their disease through disease management interventions can be shown by repeated measurements over time. If results are unsatisfactory, new avenues of patient education can be implemented, including detailed written information, disease-specific classes for instructions, reference materials on CD-ROM for computer display, or videotapes with disease-specific information.

Provider Knowledge

Physicians, physicians' assistants, and nurse practitioners are assumed to be very knowledgeable about the disease conditions that their patients face. In practice, provider knowledge of specific diseases and their diagnosis and treatment is highly variable. It is dependent on multiple factors, such as the practitioner's level of interest in the disease, volume of patients seen with the condition, reading of medical texts or best-practice materials, and participation in continuing medical education seminars.

Disease management interventions will enable practitioners to standardize their practice patterns for a given condition around a practice guideline or best-practice recommendation and to learn more about the current treatment of the disease condition. Some of these recommendations will be new knowledge to the caregiver.

Disease-specific gain of knowledge by a practitioner can be directly measured before the implementation of a disease management program and later at a standard time after the program is well established. It would be expected that baseline levels of knowledge of a particular disease might be highly variable before the disease management intervention but that the later survey would show higher and more uniform levels of disease-specific knowledge. The difference in knowledge between the practitioner surveys is the incremental disease-specific knowledge arising from the implementation of the disease management intervention.

Outcomes Measures

Mortality

Clinical outcomes are measured differences in the health status of patients after the provision of health care services. As this definition would imply, clinical outcomes are multidimensional, representing many possible measures of health status. The easiest clinical outcome to understand is the death of the patient. Death is a final and unequivocal outcome, if we disregard the legalistic difference between brain death in a patient with a living body and the total death of all organ systems of the body. Mortality is routinely observed and recorded, lending itself to be a widely used measure of clinical outcomes.

But death has its variants, which complicate the use of raw mortality data as a measure of comparative performance. Some patients have expected deaths in expected locations of care (eg, terminal cancer patients may die in a hospice). The high mortality rate of a hospice is expected. Patients with terminal diseases and physician's orders not to resuscitate (DNR) may die of a bacterial pneumonia in a hospital setting, an expected outcome for the physician and the family.

The epidemiology of death limits its widespread use. Most patients who die are elderly or very young. Death is rare enough in people between ages 1 to 50 years to make the measure impossible to use as a comparative measure, unless the population under analysis is very large (over 500,000 people).

Comparative mortality rates are useful in patients with common acute conditions that have relatively high death rates associated with the underlying disease. Examples are bacterial pneumonia, thrombotic stroke, and pulmonary emboli. Similarly, surgical procedures that have a high mortality rate associated with them can be compared by using mortality rates. Examples are coronary artery bypass surgery (CABG) for ischemic heart disease, cardiac transplant surgery, and surgery for cranial arteriovenous malformations. Adequate case mix and severity mix adjustments are a necessary preparation for the use of comparative mortality measures of outcomes. Raw mortality rates, without case mix or severity mix adjustment, will be dismissed by practitioners as meaningless.

Morbidity

Morbidity is a measure of the worsening of the patient's clinical condition after the patient has received health care services or while he or she is in a health care setting before definitive treatment. Morbidity is most easily measured by serial laboratory tests (decreasing renal function, progressive anemia), repeated physical examination (enlarging liver size, greater pedal edema), and trending of vital signs (higher fever, faster respiratory rate). The measures of morbidity may be generic, as in progressive, multiple organ failure from sepsis or any other cause, or may be disease specific, as in falling arterial blood gas levels from pneumonia.

The advantage of morbidity as a comparative measure of clinical outcomes is in its prevalence. Morbidity levels change frequently in many patients, and much more commonly than the rate of patient death. Thus, smaller numbers of patients are needed to demonstrate a measurable difference in performance.

The disadvantages in the use of morbidity measures are the degree of difficulty in accessing the underlying data elements. Physical examination data are recorded in physicians' notes, vital signs in nurses' notes, and laboratory data in the laboratory section of a medical record (which may be computerized by laboratory information systems). Consequently, most morbidity data need to be manually extracted from a patient's medical record, an expensive process requiring skilled abstractors searching for defined data elements with precise definitions of the required data to be abstracted.

Code-based measures of morbidity are available from ICD-9 codes, such as renal failure, oliguria, or hypotension. The advantage of their easy access in electronic format is balanced against the realistic concerns that these codes may not be commonly applied in patients who fit the morbidity definitions. An organization with few coded morbidities may be favorably compared to one with more accurate diagnostic coding. Further, the completeness of diagnostic coding may be limited by incomplete training and familiarity of the coding personnel with the available ICD-9 codes for morbidity measures. These are appropriate cautions in the use of code-based measures of morbidity.

Complications

Complications are unfavorable clinical consequences of diagnostic or therapeutic procedures. Examples are allergic reactions to radiologic contrast materials, postoperative hemorrhages or infections, and dehiscence of surgical wounds.

Complications are good measures of clinical outcomes, since they usually reflect breakdowns of the processes of care that give rise to the specific complication. In theory, the more incomplete and variable the procedure of care is, the more common the complication rate after the procedure. One would expect the highest complication rates to be associated with the worst processes of care.

Complications are normally documented in the medical record and should appear in diagnostic codes on patients' billing documents. But, as in the case of morbidity, there are realistic concerns that the prevalence and accuracy of codes of patient complications are not complete.[7]

Self-Assessed Functional Status and Quality of Life

Gains in patients' functional status and quality of life represent definite improvements in clinical status and outcomes. These results may be attributable to specific disease management interventions. Individual patients will report their changed perceptions of their functional status and abilities to perform activities of daily living. They also may give the relative ranking of the functional capabilities that are the most important to them. To a large extent, patients' sense of contentment or well-being is formed by their ability to participate in those activities that they most treasure, whether intellectual, physical, recreational, or avocational. Gains in functional status are not enough but must be matched with those capabilities most desired by individual patients.[8]

Assessing the functional status of a population is much more difficult than assessing that of a group of patients with a known condition. More surveys must be sent out and collected. A more generic survey must be employed, since the infirmities of the population as a whole and of the individual patient are not known. Patients' utility functions of their functional capacities are more diverse and harder to aggregate in a population-based measure.

Baseline self-assessment of a population is useful to assess the disease mix, risk mix, and public health levels of that population. Smaller cohorts of the populations can be identified for disease-specific interventions. Comparison of different populations will show different opportunities for patient education and self-care. Incremental gains in functional status for an entire population are desirable but are hard to attribute to one cause, such as a disease management intervention for a subpopulation.

Issues in the Continuous Production of Outcomes Measures

Tracking and Trending of Outcome Measures

Once critical measures of success are selected, they should be consistently produced for monitoring of performance and management of the disease management initiative. Critical measures should be consistently used over time. Only in this fashion can performance be reliably compared over sequential time periods.

The most easily understood display of process or outcomes measures over time is in the graphical form of a trend line report, tracking one or more measures across multiple time periods, frequently in monthly or quarterly increments. Such data displays allow easy visual comprehension of the performance trends by almost all observers.

Thresholds of Optimum Performance

What is the level of acceptable performance? Is it a level parallel to the average level of performance, measured over historical time periods? One can achieve this goal simply by preventing the current level of performance from deteriorating, not a very challenging goal. Is it a level that matches, or even surpasses, the levels of performance of external best-of-class systems for which performance results are available? Such results, while highly desirable, might be unachievable, certainly over the short term.

Physician managers may select different performance thresholds to be achieved at set milestones in the disease management implementation. Such a strategy will allow early successes and will facilitate team building and greater morale, yet will still permit greater levels of performance to be expected and achieved over longer time periods.

Measures of Uncertainty, Standard Deviation, and Trim Points

With any trending of performance levels, normal process variation will occur, causing upward and downward deflections of performance levels. In a disease management system with stable processes, this normal variation may be expressed as standard deviations from the mean (average) level of performance. If the processes are subject to random variation, two standard deviations from the mean will enclose 95% of the observed measures of performance. Extraordinary causes of process variation will cause the trend line to show excess variation in outcome levels beyond two standard deviations from the mean.

Physician managers must first determine the extent to which the processes in their disease management system are stable and "in control." If they are out of process control, trend measures of performance will be highly erratic, frequently reversing direction and easily passing through expected statistical barriers at plus or minus two standard deviations from the mean. No process improvement or outcomes performance improvement can be expected from disease management systems outside consistent processes of care. The first priority is to create stable and consistent processes of care across the disease management system. Only then can the processes of care be changed with the expectation that superior processes of care will achieve higher levels of performance.

With stable production systems, trim points can be created in trend reports to show differences in performance levels that are important to medical managers.

Such trim points do not have to be at levels of statistical significance from the norm. A 90% reduction in postoperative complications may be very important to medical managers but not statistically significant from historical levels of complications. Conversely, a medical manager does not have to wait for a 90% increase in complications to become statistically significant before corrective action is taken.

Modeling of Opportunity Costs, Cost Savings, and Clinical Results

Measurement of performance results of disease management systems is the first step in a more complicated endeavor requiring intimate knowledge of the processes of care, the critical process steps that drive differences in resource utilization and clinical outcomes, and the acceptable levels of process variation at each step of the health care delivery process. This is a process of modeling the disease management system to determine the investments required to create and improve the disease management interventions. For each different disease to be managed, a different investment will be required, with different results in cost savings (or investments) and clinical results. The opportunity costs are the alternative uses of the invested money and managerial effort.

CONCLUSION

The production of critical outcomes measures is crucial to the management of disease management initiatives. As described in this chapter, the construction and production of key outcomes measures is an arduous and challenging endeavor. But, seen from the perspective of the steps of data collection, analysis of the assembled data, and production of the desired outcome measures, the process can be understood and planned, and the key outcome measures can be produced. Only through an analysis of the results of health care interventions can the processes of care be rationalized and improved. This is the paramount professional challenge to the physician executive who has the responsibility to execute a carefully planned and successful disease management program.

The science and technology of outcomes measurement and management will be advanced only if the pioneers describe and publish their methods and results, both favorable and unfavorable. From such publicly available experience, a series of outcome measures might be considered as "standards" for comparison and profiling of disease management programs. The role of the physician executive in shaping and managing the diverse technologies of outcomes management cannot be overstated. For physicians truly interested in improving patient care and the systems that deliver health care, there can be no higher calling.

References

1. *A Guide to Designing a Diabetes Outcomes Measurement System: A Practical Guide for Managed Care Organizations.* Santa Monica, Calif: Value Health Sciences; 1996. Internal document.

2. Winslow R. Doctors lack practice in angioplasty. *Wall Street Journal.* November 14, 1996: B1, B6.

3. Knaus WA, Draper EA, Wagner DP, Zimmerman JE. An evaluation of outcome from intensive care in major medical centers. *Ann Intern Med.* 1986;104:410–418.

4. Hannan EL, Kilburn H Jr, O'Donnell JF, Lukacik G, Shields EP. Adult open heart surgery in New York State: an analysis of risk factors and hospital mortality rates. *JAMA.* 1990;264:2768–2774.

5. Ware JE Jr, Sherbourne CD. The MOS 36-Item Short-Form Health Survey (SF-36). 1. Conceptual framework and item selection. *Med Care.* 1992;30:473–483.

6. Ware JE, Bayliss MS, Rogers WH, et al. Differences in 4-year health outcomes for elderly and poor, chronically ill patients treated in HMO and fee-for-service systems: results from the Medical Outcomes Study. *JAMA.* 1996;276:1039–1047.

7. Iezzoni LI, Foley SM, Daley J, Hughes J, Fisher ES, Heeren T. Comorbidities, complications, and coding bias: does the number of diagnosis codes matter in predicting in-hospital mortality? *JAMA.* 1992;267:2197–2203.

8. Stewart AL, Greenfield S, Hays RD, et al. Functional status and well-being of patients with chronic conditions: results from the Medical Outcomes Study. JAMA. 1989;262:907–913. Erratum, *JAMA.* 1989;262:2542.

CHAPTER 5

Information Systems for Disease Management

David J. Brailer and Jason Dandridge

As health care providers respond to the call for greater efficiency in health care delivery, the management of patients on a disease-specific basis has emerged as a way to provide care closely tailored to the manifestations and treatment of specific diseases. This transformation in care delivery has driven important changes in the way information is collected, analyzed, and used in health care. Both the efficiency of care and the specialization of care to a specific disease require information that is more current, comprehensive, and accurate than that previously required for billing and related tasks. The advent of firms specializing in disease management and the implementation of disease management initiatives by the full range of participants in health care delivery has spawned new demands on information technology. Disease management entities are investing heavily in information systems and data collection vehicles as part of their efforts to tightly manage the care process and to satisfy the information support needs of their many stakeholders.

Focusing as it does on specific diseases rather than on market segments (e.g., health maintenance organizations [HMOs]), care technologies (e.g., imaging), care processes (e.g., surgical procedures), or a single stakeholder (e.g., employers), disease management necessarily straddles the needs of many market elements. It is the job of disease management to incorporate the views of various stakeholders and forge a common vision for clinical delivery. Of the many parties involved in disease management, the four principal stakeholders are (1) institutional and product providers (hospitals and other facilities, along with drug, device, and other health care suppliers), (2) physicians and other caregivers, (3) patients, and (4) employers and other purchasers of health care services. The complementary and conflicting needs of these stakeholders are the essential forces shaping disease management and the information technology that supports it.

Providers in institutional settings need to manage the flow of patients through their facilities and ensure that human resources, physical capacity, and inventory are readily available and well utilized. Drug, device, and other health care suppliers need to optimize the value of the compounds and objects they manufacture, especially to managed-care buyers, who look across whole populations. Physicians need information support that helps them determine how they can best care for any particular patient and improve their care practices. To serve their patients' needs better, they also need less cumbersome processes for ordering tests, making referrals, and finding results. At the same time, patients have to be educated on the detection and management of illness and given tools to help them understand and navigate the health delivery system. They need assurance that their symptoms and satisfaction are being given full weight in the care process. Employers need evidence that they are getting a good value for their health care expenditures. They want a process that will make it simpler for employees to switch plans or providers and that will enable them to monitor the delivery of services to employees without having to be too involved in day-to-day details.

Each stakeholder in the disease management process has a unique and different perspective that affects the process of gathering information, the type of information collected, and its use. Stakeholders may agree to common access only to certain data (e.g., data concerning access or patient education). The use of other data sought by two or three stakeholders may be resisted by another stakeholder (e.g., providers may resist providing quality data to employers/purchasers and patients). In some instances, stakeholders may all require information that is particular to their own needs. These data may be irrelevant to or even in conflict with other stakeholder needs. The detailed clinical data that health plans want about patients to stratify premiums across populations on the basis of their relative health status and risk of adverse outcomes would be an example.

Even when there is agreement on what information is to be collected and how it is to be used, different stakeholders place different values on various elements of information and therefore invest differently in collection. For example, functional status information requires the patient to do extra work (i.e., filling out the survey) and the provider to bear extra cost (if it collects the data). However, these data are of the most benefit to employers/purchasers, who can use them to monitor clinical effectiveness and to improve contracting with health plans. Disease management entities face challenges of similar magnitude as they try to allocate finite information technology budgets across a broad diversity of interests. Each stakeholder can have a myopic view of the entire disease process. It is therefore essential that the disease manager determine how to meet the information needs of each stakeholder as part of the overall business plan. The successful utilization of data for disease management requires attention to all stakeholders.

This chapter is intended as a guide for those who are designing disease management information systems or using them as inputs into their disease management programs. It reviews the needs of the four primary stakeholder groups and how these translate into information investments and presents an overview of the seven core information technologies that constitute the bulk of systems that support disease management: (1) clinical information systems and data repositories, (2) data integration, (3) electronic medical records, (4) decision-support and expert systems, (5) practice management systems, (6) community health information networks, and (7) the Internet and Intranets. It also proposes an information system development and implementation strategy that translates disease management program goals into the overall design of an information system and an implementation process. It concludes with a set of practices for implementing information technology solutions and selecting third-party vendors and products.

The chapter emphasizes three principles that should help the reader identify and avoid the most costly mistakes of information systems deployment. First, the business plan for the disease management entity must clearly articulate how the information technology relates to achievement of the business purpose of the organization. If the organization's business plan fails to address this clearly, successful information system implementation is unlikely. Second, information technology implementation should be incremental and successful at each step. Many organizations commit to implementing large-scale, monolithic information systems, but this is a risky and lengthy process that often lags behind the short-lived business cycle of the volatile health care market. Incremental implementation ensures that each step produces net value. Though less hyperbolic than a "big bang" rollout, it reduces risk to the information strategy and the organization. Third, one must demonstrate that the investment in information technology creates a positive return on investment for one or more stakeholders. In information technology investment decisions, positive return on investment does not exclude intangible benefits that justify the cost (i.e., improved quality of care or ability to remain competitive), provided that the decision maker determines that the benefits— however these are measured—can be shown to outweigh the fully laden costs of information technology investments. Those who apply these principles will be able to deliver more reliable, successful, and profitable information technology— and hence disease management—than those who do not. That is the essence of this chapter.

DISEASE MANAGEMENT INFORMATION STRATEGY

The core business strategy of disease management is to provide comprehensive, multisite care across the lifetime of health and illness for a subpopulation defined by having, having had, or being at risk for a specific disease. Disease management has the capacity to enhance clinical and service quality as well as the efficiency of care delivery. The essential role of information technology in disease management is to assemble all relevant data, from every facility and the home, about patients with or at risk for a disease and to use the data to engage the provider, physician, patient, and employer in a less expensive, higher-quality care delivery process.

This challenge is simple to state, but it is complicated, costly, and risky to meet. The information technology for disease management must perform many tasks: assembling available data, collecting data heretofore unavailable, housing the data for efficient access, identifying and tracking specific patients across many facilities and years through unique identification codes, rendering the data into rigorous and valid information, and presenting data to users in meaningful ways for a variety of uses. Prioritizing and sequencing these tasks means making trade-offs across stakeholders (listed and described in Table 5–1) and narrowing the "value proposition" of disease management to that which can be supported by affordable information technology.

To be viable, disease management must transform the ways providers, physicians, patients, and employers perform their respective disease-related tasks and the ways they all interact. This is why information technology must go beyond collecting, manipulating, and displaying information. It must accomplish the core business strategy for the entity concerned with disease management by shifting the role and behavior of each stakeholder.

Table 5–1 Disease Management Stakeholders

Stakeholder	Description
Institutional and product providers	Institutions or organizations that provide care to patients (e.g., hospitals, physician practices, and nursing homes) and that make devices and products used by patients (e.g., drug makers)
Physicians and other caregivers	Individuals who provide health care to patients (e.g., physicians, nurses, and emergency medical technicians)
Members and patients	Individuals who belong to care organizations or receive health care
Employers and purchasers	Organizations that employ those who receive health care or entities that purchase care services for their members

Providers must transform their business from one emphasizing vertical, department-based, revenue-producing care delivery into one emphasizing patient-centered, cost-minimizing, cross-continuum integration of clinical services. Physicians and other caregivers need information systems to become care process managers who spend their time making informed judgments about alternative therapies and delivering care rather than collecting data and being fact finders. This management of the care process is a key feature in the improvement of clinical performance. For their part, patients must become partners in the care process by using data to make better self- or provider-delivered treatment decisions. After decades of acculturation to a passive role, patients are now being asked to become informed, self-directed coworkers in disease management. Some patients will embrace this role, whereas others will be insecure in it, but all will need accessible information and guidance on how to use it. Finally, employers must reinvent themselves from myopic bottom-line contracting organizations into organizations that direct care to the providers and physicians who demonstrate their superior value and their comfort with the new shape of health care delivery. All stakeholders will be improved by the disease management information system, but only if they use the information to alter their historical practices.

Many organizations within the health care industry have made substantial improvements in their ability to deliver timely, relevant information to stakeholders at the required locations. This has been accomplished primarily through the judicious use of seven core technologies to achieve business goals. These core technologies serve different purposes and perform different functions, but all have been created to improve information flow and access. Table 5–2 lists the seven core technologies and provides a brief description of each.

Institutional and Product Providers

Hospital providers and health plans have undergone significant change in their business operations over the past few years as they have responded to the threat of reduction of traditional revenue sources such as indemnity-based fee-for-service payments and discounts. They are also redefining their market role by taking risks and becoming full-spectrum disease managers. Providers are moving from being "rent-free workshops"[1] to full-scale organizations with three components: financing, delivery systems, and care management. Disease management fits into all three components of this strategy but has particular resonance for delivery systems and care management.

From a delivery systems perspective, providers are using information systems to lower their administrative costs by reducing excess capacity and redundant services. As they manage diseases, the goal becomes one of balancing capacity across related sites of care rather than optimizing capacity utilization at a single site (e.g., "all beds full"). This requires substantial information about the demand

Table 5–2 Core Technologies

Core Technology	Description
Clinical information systems (CISs) and data repositories	Systems that capture and store objective and subjective medical data such as physician and patient observations, risk factors, test orders and results, treatments provided, vital signs, and procedures performed
Data integration	An activity or concept in which different data sources and/or systems are linked or combined to facilitate the sharing of data, reduce data inconsistencies, improve data accuracy, improve data integrity, and create a more integrated information environment
Electronic medical records (EMRs)	Distributed electronic systems that provide and capture necessary medical and patient information at the point of care
Decision-support systems (DSSs) and expert systems (ESs)	Systems that use information to help stakeholders make better decisions or that use rules, expert knowledge, and information to offer solutions to problems
Practice management systems (PMSs)	Systems that allow physician practices to manage day-to-day operational activities such as billing, scheduling, and electronic communication. In addition, they aid physicians in decision making by providing access to medical information such as population research and laboratory data
Community health information networks (CHINs)	Traditionally, electronic networks that link all of the stakeholders in a particular geographic region to facilitate shared information. However, more recently, CHINs have moved toward more content-focused rather than technology-focused groups seeking to address their communities' health information needs.
Internet and Intranets	Electronic external or internal infrastructure that provides communication among and information access to all stakeholders

behavior of disease in various settings, along with empirical data showing how this can be modified by interventions such as patient education and financial incentives. For the delivery system that has widespread operations and multiple entities that are quasi-related, information technology holds the promise of reducing redundant services such as hospital admissions for chest pain (when an abnormal electrocardiogram reflects no change in the patient's condition but the baseline is in another facility), imaging (when a specialist consults on a disease process and must repeat key imaging studies because they will take too long to transfer and the patient is ill), or laboratory tests for cholesterol (routinely performed but infrequently needed). These areas do not involve clinical decision making per se, but rather how administrative operations translate clinical orders into systemwide actions.

Likewise, health plans have sought to reduce the administrative cost of their operations by reducing the cost of data collection, utilization review, and network development. Health plans are managing diseases by instituting demand management centers that give them direct access to patients, separate and apart from the primary care physician. These centers make referral decisions, monitor care, and provide education. The data they collect are useful in evaluating the efficacy of services offered by the health plan as well as the performance of providers and physicians. These data are critical to their contracting and development of value to purchasers in key disease areas. As health plans become more like true provider organizations in managing the delivery of clinical services, their needs for widely dispersed, clinically integrated data will match those of any provider.

In a departure from their historical laissez-faire approach to care process management, providers are beginning to see the market and financial benefits of an activist approach to this task. In many provider organizations, disease management is equated with the choice to integrate facilities and delivery processes across the spectrum of care. Though provider institutions have been the location and frequently the source of care delivery, they have largely abstained from managing the care process. However, as providers merge or enter into joint ventures with finance and insurance companies and as health plans step up their medical management activities, providers have become more willing to address issues of clinical process—test usage, therapeutic alternatives, complication reduction, and patient flow management. They have seized care management as a key means of differentiating their services and of gaining a competitive advantage over each other.

In the short run, the disease-managing provider faces the nagging problem of harming intensity-based revenue (fee-for-service–like payments), since care management inevitably leads to a reduction of billable services. This creates dissonance over the degree to which the organization should embrace a risk-taking, cost-cutting business strategy to position itself for the future. The ambiguity is represented in the information strategy of the provider organization. Not surprisingly, since the two business strategies are in conflict, the priorities for information systems investment and the expectations of information systems are confused. To maximize profitability under intensity-based payments, billing, contract management, and market share management information is needed. Tools such as clinical integration or outcomes measurement systems are simply cost increasing unless they enhance billing yield. Under a full-risk approach, the tools for care process management have value because they facilitate care process management. Disease management allows providers to implement future-oriented business strategies while maintaining present-day profitability.

Other "providers" who have a stake in the delivery process—pharmaceutical, device, and other health care suppliers—are reexamining their core strategies and finding that their new business models are markedly different from those of the past in ways that have substantial implications for information technology. Historically, these providers needed nothing more than relatively simple information tools—simple spreadsheet or database technologies, marketing databases, advertising yield assessment tools, and clinical trial management tools—to conduct their nonmanufacturing business. The buyer did not have to justify the business value of devices and supplies, ranging from new drugs to new surgical tools to imaging equipment.

Pharmaceutical, device, and health care supply companies, like institutional providers, find it difficult to turn away from their historically simple, profitable business model to a model of risk taking and disease management. Disease management has to date meant developing different ways of marketing products to meet traditional goals, not a fundamental shift in goals. It now reflects the recognition that health care must sell its output to various decision makers who buy on behalf of numerous users rather than engaging in point-to-point selling. These buyers look for cost-benefit analyses, efficacy studies, and heavy review of data in making decisions. As the market shifts toward full risk sharing, they will face the same fundamental choice as institutional providers: when to shift their core business model, and hence their information strategy, to full risk acceptance. In this case, they must approach their business as a manager of an aspect of the care process and must provide the full spectrum of services, information tools, drugs, and devices required for a disease area or a market sector. Thus, a maker of intensive care unit (ICU) drugs might also supply ICU monitoring equipment and advanced cardiac management education technology. A chemotherapy manufacturer might manage a cancer care delivery organization with specialized information tools (such as Zeneca Pharmaceuticals in alliance with Salick Health Care).

Four technologies constitute the key elements of information systems used by providers and health care suppliers for disease management. The first is clinical information systems and data repositories. These are vital to providers' ability to track specific patients over time and to create normative databases that can be used for widespread system management or for heavily specialized settings (e.g., the ICU). The second is data integration and electronic data interchange, which is the ability to assemble disparate financial, clinical, operational, and strategic data in real time and to provide concurrent responses to new findings. The third is practice management systems. These first three tools provide the backbone connection between physicians in practice and allow the clinical delivery system to function on a virtual basis. The fourth tool is the Internet and Intranets. As with every aspect of disease management technology, the Internet and Intranets are rapidly transforming how services and organizations are integrated and how they relate to the outside market.

Physicians and Other Caregivers

Economically, physicians have generally sought to maintain a balance between their incomes and the time they must devote to their practices. Organizationally, physicians have long been stand-alone, semipassive participants in the affairs of the delivery system outside their own office or preferred hospital. Historically, they have cared for their patients; signed up with nearly every independent practice association (IPA), HMO, and physician hospital organization (PHO) that sought their participation; and referred patients to their trusted peers. Clinically, physicians have placed the reasoning associated with clinical decision making on a near-sacred level. At the same time, they have been frustrated by the boredom of mundane workups and treatments that have not changed in years. These forces have had a substantial impact on the development of information systems for physicians. Physicians have not been willing to use information systems at the bedside or in the clinic because of justifiable fears of slowing the throughput of patients, despite evidence that these systems improve the quality and lower the overall cost of care. Likewise, physicians have not used therapeutic decision-support tools that optimize application of treatment regimens because of inconvenience, impracticality, and inaccuracy, among other reasons. Even in the seemingly simple area of practice automation, physicians have been largely unwilling to use tools that are linked to a given payer because of the wide diversity of payers with whom they contract. These forces have made physicians neutral toward information systems, although some may be antagonistic.

The emergence of disease management and numerous other forces have reshaped the work of physicians and the way they use information technology. At the same time, noteworthy advances in clinical tools—knowledge bases, decision-support algorithms, user interface technology, and detailed clinical databases—have brought to the threshold of acceptability information tools that physicians can use. These technologies enable physicians to play a dual role in patient care. At the patient level, the decision-support tools intersect with the physician's judgment to navigate patients through the multiple, competing alternative therapies or approaches. At the organization level, they assist the physician or a designated leader or physician executive with the determination of the policies that govern the delivery of clinical care for a delivery system. These roles are not mutually exclusive. They are drawn from an important principle of bringing information technologies to physicians. They invest in technologies that help the physician manage the patient better and with less time and effort. They invest in systems that give the physician a broader view of the way patients are being cared for in general.

Among physicians who manage disease areas (specialists, procedural physicians, and certain primary care physicians such as obstetricians), there has been a groundswell of demand for the kind of information that will help them better treat their patients. They currently spend a large percentage of their time reassembling and interpreting basic information collected in the primary care setting. Numerous data elements required for disease-specific care that are not collected by primary care physicians must be gathered. Correspondence with primary care physicians is often slow, noninteractive, and subject to communication failures. The information collected by disease management efforts has the potential to improve and simplify these physicians' efforts. Data collected in the primary care setting can be available to them during care encounters, and their own findings and recommendations can be made available to primary care physicians immediately and interactively.

Three key technologies will be core elements in transforming physician practices. The first is electronic medical records and their closely related counterparts, computerized medical records. These tools will bring together detailed patient information that can be used to manage a patient in real time, along with problem lists, formularies, and other supplemental data. Although physicians have been reluctant to use computer technology in their relationship with patients, the benefits that these bring in reducing data collection time, allowing portability of data across practitioners and sites of care, and bringing basic information to concurrent decision making will offset the time demands and inconvenience that many physicians will encounter in using them. A small segment of (mostly) younger, computer-literate physicians will undoubtedly use these tools.

The second technology is decision-support systems and expert systems, which can improve the quality of clinical decision making, reduce the turnaround time for decisions, provide a pattern of decisions for many physicians, and prevent clinical errors (e.g., drug-drug interactions). These benefits will bring important benefits to disease areas where most physicians do not frequently provide care and to the typical disease, where established norms of practice interfere with efforts to improve clinical performance. The third technology is the Internet and Intranets, which will allow physicians to gain access to clinical knowledge, treatment protocols, databases, and patient data from a single source, regardless of the location or type of computer.

Members and Patients

The role of patients in their own care is undergoing substantial revision. Under the traditional insurance coverages in effect over the past 50 years, patients were discouraged from questioning the nature or quality of the care they received. Although they could tell good care from bad, so long as they were not too ill to judge the quality of care, for the most part they became passive participants in their own care. Even educated patients became passive in care decisions. Moreover, the health care system effectively forced many underinformed patients—those most likely to neglect preventive care—into delaying treatment and using emergency and other acute services in lieu of other more appropriate sites of care. The new health care paradigm calls for patients to be coproducers of their care rather than merely recipients of services. The positive results achieved through the active self-education of patients with cancer, AIDS, and many chronic diseases have proven the value of this interaction. Further proof of the capacity of patients to be active participants in the delivery system can be found in the intensifed advocacy on behalf of ill children, enrollment switches across HMOs, the Federal Employees Health Benefits Plan, and the use of family medical guides and other information sources.

Disease management relies upon patients who are active in three areas of care: management of illness, delivery of self-care, and making informed choices about alternative therapies, providers, or physicians. Patient participation in management of care includes scheduling appointments with primary care physicians and specialists, scheduling preventive care and screening, switching physicians and other health plans, and planning for terminal care. Patient self-care areas largely include using over-the-counter medications and seeking child care. Informed choice activities include examining cost and outcome profiles for physicians and hospitals, participation in disease-specific education forums, and understanding end-of-life options for care (e.g., hospice, treatment versus no treatment). Information technology has traditionally been unable to help patients and members with these tasks, but as technology evolves and patients become more engaged in disease management programs, the number of tasks assisting patients by technology (e.g., scheduling an appointment over the Internet) will increase.

The prospect of active patients calls attention to the deepest shift in the health care market that disease management captures: the emerging role of consumerism in health care services. Although the sophistication of the patient is typically low, it is increasing steadily. Generational shifts will bring substantial change. Programs that include patient empowerment in their business strategy and invest in the information systems to engage the patient will be well positioned to take advantage of this shift. Accordingly, the technology needed to support patient empowerment must overcome several constraints. First, it must be useful to someone with no technical training and with limited education. Second, it must be available in the home, the workplace, and the physician's office or provider setting. Third, the marginal cost of operation must be low. Fourth, it must be generic across physicians, health plans, or providers.

Current technologies that meet these criteria include cable television, videotapes, interactive videodisk, interactive telephone, computer programs, Internet services, published books, CD-ROM, and radio. Not surprisingly, the media that play the largest role in the general affairs of the public also are the most commonly used forms of patient empowerment in health care delivery. As the media industries consolidate and evolve, multimedia services on fixed media (e.g., CD-ROM) and networked media (e.g., Internet or cable modem) will become prominent means of giving patients the information they want and need as active participants in disease management services. Of mounting interest is the Internet and its ability to present compact, education- and demographic-tailored, current information to any household.

Employers and Purchasers

Employers and other purchasers of care are often ambivalent about their role in the delivery of health care services for their employees. On one hand, they are deeply concerned about the cost of health care within their compensation plans. On the other hand, they are reluctant to depart from the strongly held view (with a few exceptions) that managing health care is not the core competence of their businesses. Employers are divided on disease management. Some see it as one of several often futile attempts to control health care costs. Others see it as a starting point for them to engage directly in the health management process.

A fundamental question for employers is whether they see procurement of health care services as a core input into their businesses. Their expectations for information technology will vary with their desired roles. Those who take an activist role will desire performance information about providers and physicians, eligibility management tools, self-education systems for their employees, and utilization monitoring and management tools. Those who see health care as a cost area but not as something that the employer should manage need at a minimum performance and contracting information to deal with health plans.

Regardless of their level of activism, the overwhelming majority of employers and other purchasers will want to see factual demonstration of the value of the programs and initiatives they purchase to manage diseases, prevent downstream illness, manage utilization, and educate employees. They will want to ease the difficulties encountered by their employees in enrolling and switching plans. Information technology that collects data and can demonstrate the value of these interventions will be exceedingly valuable to the disease manager.

The two key technologies for the employer and purchaser are (1) community health information networks, which provide regional master indexes of the population and the ability to automate data transfer and enrollment; and (2) Internet and Intranet technologies, which can benefit the communications and monitoring activities of employers as they do every other stakeholder in disease management.

CORE TECHNOLOGIES

Each of the four stakeholders in disease management requires one or more of the seven information technologies that are central to information technology investments in disease management (see Table 5–2). Many of these applications, such as clinical information systems (CISs) and electronic medical records (EMRs), can add value to and improve the quality of disease management. However, the role of information technology in disease management is simply an extension of its general role in the health care system. An EMR, for example, has the potential to vastly improve disease management and decision making by providing the caregiver with longitudinal patient information at the point of care (POC). However, an EMR system should also be implemented as part of a greater enterprise-wide initiative to improve the quality of care in all areas of health care delivery. Consequently, disease management is not likely to provide the impetus for implementing information technology, but rather should be one of its many beneficiaries. Similarly, if an organization recognizes that its infrastructure does not include a specific information technology application that could improve disease management, a more fundamental and strategic issue must be addressed. The entity must consider not only how disease management could be improved, but how its overall management of health care delivery could be enhanced with the introduction of that information technology solution.

The distinctions among the information technology applications can be obscured in some cases due to the different capabilities that can be included in each. For example, an EMR can be designed to include decision-support capabilities. A stand-alone decision-support system (DSS) can be developed and accessed separately. Regardless of the lines drawn between the different components of the information technology infrastructure, each application must be integrated with the others to provide the necessary information and meet the functionality objectives for improved management of disease.

Each of the core technologies can play an important role in improving disease management. However, these technologies are most beneficial when they are used in conjunction with one another to produce an information and technological infrastructure that delivers necessary information to stakeholders at required locations. Therefore, a disease management entity should evaluate the potential benefit of the core technologies and determine which to use and how to use them together to accomplish business objectives. Figure 5–1 provides an example of an information technology infrastructure for a disease management entity. This example demonstrates how different core technologies might be used to provide information to stakeholders. An important point to recognize is that each of the stakeholders has access to relevant information necessary to improve the overall quality and effectiveness of disease management.

Clinical Information Systems and Data Repositories

Historically, in addition to financial and accounting systems, clinical information systems (CISs) have been at the core of health care delivery. These systems capture objective and subjective medical data such as physician and patient observations, risk factors, test orders and results, treatment provided, vital signs, and procedures performed.[2,3] The original driver for developing CISs was to reduce the costs of health care services by gathering information to permit more informed decisions. Overall, providers have been successful at achieving the first goal: gathering information, one of the key enablers of disease management.

Many organizations that have gathered clinical data for many years have a store of information that can be used to manage diseases better. These systems often contain longitudinal information that can identify treatments that have been most successful for a disease and can isolate population trends over time. This information has the potential to give caregivers and providers better insight into the manifestations of diseases, a deeper understanding of the costs for diagnosing those diseases, and an enhanced knowledge of how to manage those diseases more effectively and efficiently. In addition, this information has the potential to improve payers' ability to manage costs and contract with the lowest-cost, yet highest-quality, providers.

These potential benefits of CISs have yet to be recognized in most organizations. Few have been able to organize and use the collected data. Though CISs have generally been successful in capturing clinical data, the data have often been inaccurate and incomplete because they have not been seen as a care process management tool. In addition, providers have not been able to transform the data into information that can be interpreted and used in decision making. In many provider organizations, CISs have become huge data dumps—an electronic method of storing information that used to be warehoused in huge paper file rooms. However, the ability to access and aggregate that data is not significantly greater than it was in the days of the paper file room.

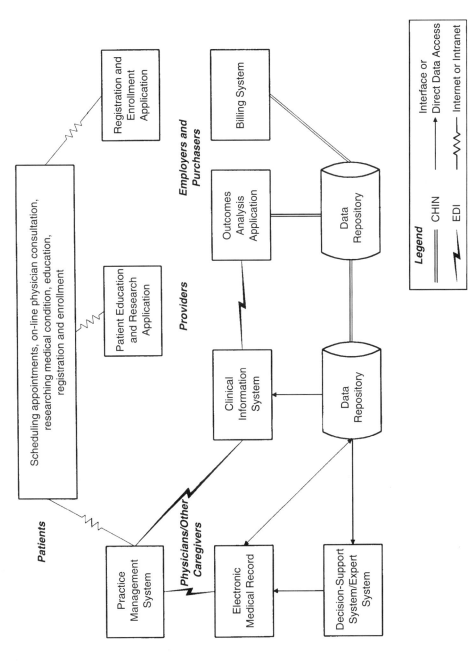

Figure 5-1 Disease Management Information Flow

Data accuracy, completeness, and accessibility have been recurring problems with CISs, primarily because the usefulness of these systems has not been sufficient to induce physicians and caregivers to make them an integral part of their care delivery processes. Many organizations are beginning to implement graphical user interfaces (GUIs) as more useful covers to the often uninteresting and uninviting mainframe screens, but the input mechanisms are still not intuitively accessible to many new users.

Many caregivers do not understand how to operate the systems, what data to enter and where, and most of all, how entering this data will better their job in the future. Once the data are in the system, users find it difficult to retrieve the information in a manner that is relevant to their jobs. Physicians cannot be expected to take the time to learn a new method of operation if the direct benefit to their work has not been proven to them. These problems can be attributed to poor design and implementation of the CIS.

In addition, the point of entry for these systems is often quite inconvenient. Many hospitals still record clinical information on paper and later enter it into the CIS. But the point of entry into the system is not the same as the point of care (POC). This increases data duplication efforts, inaccurate data, and data that are not entered into the system at all.

Finally, the terminology used in these systems is often vague and inconsistent with caregivers' definitions. In many cases, these systems are developed with very little caregiver consultation. Systems developers and engineers often develop the systems with terminology that is open to interpretation. For example, a data entry field on a CIS screen may be labeled "fever." A caregiver may not know whether this field is "yes/no" or a numeric temperature. Furthermore, physicians have learned a more nuanced vocabulary and may interpret a field differently than the developers intended.

The problems that plague the successful and regular use of CISs can be resolved if proper actions are taken at the outset of the design and if the system is evaluated on an ongoing basis. A CIS will not succeed if it is developed singularly for the purpose of automating the paper file room. The business objectives of and vision for the system must be defined so that they will help drive the development process and ensure that the results add value to disease management efforts.[4]

However, defining objectives is not enough. No matter how focused the effort is on the system's purpose, if it is not usable and does not meet users' needs, the CIS will fail. To minimize this risk, end users must be highly involved in the definition and design of the system. The development process must be iterative, allowing the users to provide continual feedback. In addition, users must be sufficiently trained to understand how to use the system and, most importantly, how it can improve the quality and efficiency of their work.

Finally, after implementation, the system and its usage must be evaluated on an ongoing basis. Before the implementation, a set of measures should be defined to gauge the system's success. Once the system is in use, the measures should be used to answer questions such as whether caregivers are using the system and whether the system is meeting the intended objectives and standards of business functionality.

Data Integration

Data integration is a concept or activity that links data sources to facilitate the sharing of data; to improve data accuracy, integrity, and accessibility; and to create a more integrated information environment. To make many of the technology solutions addressed in this chapter work successfully, organizations must integrate data sources and provide access and updates to those sources from disparate locations. Disease management can be improved significantly if the quality and cost of care can be measured, controlled, and improved throughout the entire continuum of care. These activities can be performed more effectively if data sources and systems are integrated.

With data integration, providers can perform aggregate analyses on data from different sources. For example, a hospital may develop an expert system (ES) using data from the hospital's CIS and a particular department's stand-alone system (a computer system that is not linked to any others). This requires that the data be integrated in some way. There are currently many approaches to data integration. Among them are physically integrating data into a single database or repository, interfacing systems so that information from separate databases is available, and developing interface engines that support messaging across disparate databases.

Completely integrating data into a single repository is an onerous task, involving a complicated process of identifying all data elements required by all systems. Redundancies must be removed, and each of the systems must be programmed either to update this central repository in addition to its own databases or to rely solely on the single repository. This effort has been started in many organizations and is continuing in most, but success is difficult to achieve due to the long lead times involved. For example, the data dictionary (a listing of all fields contained in a database) is affected by each new system added or old system removed. In addition, it is difficult to obtain data dictionaries for many of the older, mainframe-based systems.

Another approach to data integration is to interface systems. Interfacing systems involves developing direct links between multiple systems that deliver specifically required data. An advantage to this approach is that interfaces do not need to be developed to support every data element contained in the communicating systems. The interface needs only to be able to retrieve the required data from the source system and send it to the receiving system. However, as the need for systems to share information increases, the number of interconnections grows geometrically. At some level of interfacing, the costs and complexity outweigh the benefits.

A recent solution to some of the challenges posed by the previous two approaches is the interface engine, or *integration hub and spoke model*. The fundamental purpose of the integration hub is to act as a clearinghouse for information. All systems, or spokes, send the hub information that the other systems need and retrieve from the hub the information necessary for their own uses. The hub acts as a single data repository but needs only to store the information required by each system, rather than all of the information contained in every system. In addition, if a new system is added to the network, only one interface needs to be developed if other systems require the new system's data. The new system interfaces with the hub, and the interfaces between the hub and other systems are modified so that they can retrieve the new information. This makes the administrative and maintenance requirements more manageable and reduces the initial effort required to match data elements among systems.[5]

Often, data must be integrated not only within a single location but across disparate locations. Electronic data interchange (EDI) makes this possible. One definition of EDI is "standard electronic messages conveyed from one computer to another without manual intervention."[6] EDI is based on some standard data coding format that two computers or systems understand. Through this common format, they communicate with each other. For example, to evaluate a patient's status, a physician in an ancillary office may need access not only to the data in his or her office systems but also to a hospital's CIS. If the two systems are linked via EDI, they can transfer the necessary information automatically so that both systems have the data the physician requires in either location.

Some benefits of EDI are reduced duplication of procedures and tests; a streamlined treatment process through the timely availability of data on services provided; improved capture of financial, clinical, and administrative data; and reduced exposure to fraud and abuse.[7] The major challenge of EDI implementation is identifying the standard protocol or *language* to use among the systems. As single entities develop EDI capabilities, they will have to determine the standard. As members within networks attempt to link with other members in networks, they may meet with incompatible standards. Members will have to decide on a single standard and modify all of the systems to speak that language.

Electronic Medical Records

The primary objective of the EMR is to provide single-source information at the POC. Information is useless to caregivers if it is not available when they need it. Unfortunately, many billions of dollars have been spent to develop information systems that do not have a place in caregivers' daily operations and activities. The

EMR contains longitudinal patient data; the information contained in the CIS, as discussed above; and many other data elements that a physician can quickly locate electronically.

When the EMR was originally described, it was viewed as a mechanism to automate a patient's paper chart so that an electronic record would follow the patient throughout the continuum of care. However, more recently, the health care industry has begun to recognize the EMR as an information technology solution that integrates and provides the user access to other systems and databases such as decision-support systems (DSSs) and CISs. It is also increasingly the basis for improving the overall provider work flow and operations. Therefore, the typical functionality of the EMR includes capabilities well beyond automation of paper charts.

EMRs can be developed to include a range of functions, although the Institute of Medicine has identified "gold standard" criteria. This standard recommends that EMR systems include such capabilities as providing patient problem lists, health status measures, documentation of clinical reasoning, linkages with other clinical records to provide longitudinal data, protection from unauthorized access, continuous assessment, clinical problem solving, flexibility, and expandability.[8] These functions only represent the core capabilities of EMR systems. Many of the features discussed in the following section on decision-support systems and expert systems, such as automatic reminders and alerts, are also included in some EMR systems.

The EMR is also used to link clinical service to financial and billing information. In many provider organizations, a bill is generated by collecting the different paper-based charts and orders, attaching charges to those activities, and then entering this data into a separate billing system. Since the EMR is the central point of entry for data on all services provided, these services can automatically be matched with the associated charges under different health care plans. The accuracy and timeliness of billing, and therefore the cash flow of the provider organizations, can improve considerably.

Recent advances in technology have made feasible the vision of a decentralized system accessible at the POC. With the advance of EDI, increasingly powerful and affordable hardware and software, and mobile computing such as wireless and portable devices, access to information at any location can be achieved. However, the technology is seldom the limitation for successful implementation of an EMR.

As with the other information technologies, usability is a key factor in the ultimate success of an EMR. If caregivers do not use it, the EMR will not be successful. The EMR can be an extremely intelligent and complex system, but if the physician does not like the input device that must be used at the POC, information will be lost. Therefore, a great emphasis must be placed on fulfilling the needs of users. The EMR must use readily understandable terms and easily retrieve the information in which the users are interested. A common capability of recent EMRs concerns giving a specific user the ability to create a unique view of data. The more that users can receive specific information in the format designed to meet their own needs, the more efficient their work will be, and the more accurate and complete the information entered will be. Accordingly, both before and after implementation, extensive training must be provided to ensure that the end user is comfortable with the system and recognizes the benefits of using it.

The effort must begin by defining the business objectives and requirements of the users and continue with an iterative prototyping phase during which users can evaluate the usability and benefit of the EMR. This is of special concern in selecting a predeveloped product from a vendor. If the product is purchased and implemented without intense prepurchase evaluation by the user, it will almost certainly not meet the needs of caregivers.

The availability, accuracy, and completeness of data are also issues concerning EMR implementation. If the different repositories or databases on which the EMR is based do not contain the required data, the EMR is of little value. However, if the EMR is used by caregivers, it can be a tool to populate the repositories with correct information.

An additional challenge for EMR systems is the growing need to access the system across members of a network rather than within a single entity. This requires even more systems with different data structures and coding standards to provide information through the EMR. In addition, it requires that the EMR meet the unique needs and support the unique operations of each network member.[9]

Decision-Support Systems and Expert Systems

The purpose of both decision-support systems (DSSs) and expert systems (ESs) is to help users make better, more informed decisions. Successful DSSs and ESs accomplish this by providing relevant information at the necessary time in meaningful locations. In addition, they generally aid decision makers by analyzing data and acting on it or providing alternative recommendations for the caregiver. For example, a DSS may notify a nurse that it is time to change an intravenous line to minimize infection. Similarly, given a patient's symptom and medical guidelines or rules on which to evaluate those symptoms, an ES may offer multiple diagnoses to a physician.

For purposes of this discussion, DSSs and ESs will be treated as virtually the same. There is arguably a fine line between the two types of systems: an ES in one organization may be considered a DSS in another organization. The traditional distinction between the two is that DSSs tend to provide information in a relevant way to support a user's decision. An ES tends to offer alternative solutions for the decision. However, often an organization develops something that it calls a DSS but that provides alternatives for decision making similar to an ES. The important point to remember is that both require information, rules, and guidelines to aid in the decision process.

It is also important to consider that these types of systems are not necessarily stand-alone or separate from other information technology applications. For example, an organization may create a stand-alone DSS to complete the initial interpretation of tests or images in a specific department of a hospital. However, the provider may also build that decision support directly into an EMR, or it may also develop Internet applications to provide physicians with on-line reference and research information for decision support. Decision support and expert advice can show up in many places and on many different technical platforms.

DSSs and ESs can improve the decision-making process in disease management on the basis of analysis of information, rules, and guidelines. Some of the specific uses are

- *Determination of proper drug dose and administration schedule.* Decision support can be provided to ensure that medications are administered in the proper doses and on schedule. This could improve the overall quality and control of the disease management process.
- *Executive information systems (EISs).* These types of systems can give executives more strategic views of disease and population trends, physician practices, and costs.[10]
- *Automated critiquing of physician orders.* Caregiver orders entered into a computer can automatically be critiqued for necessity and cost-effectiveness.
- *Automated warnings, reminders, and alerts.* These systems can generate reminders that certain actions should be performed by caregivers. They may also warn of potential adverse drug reactions. The importance of activities occurring in a timely manner cannot be overstated in improving quality.
- *Diagnostic aids.* Given patient symptoms and other relevant data, these systems can suggest possible diagnoses, some of which physicians may not have considered and others of which may reaffirm the physician's beliefs.

One of the critical success factors for DSSs and ESs is access to complete and accurate data. Common sources for these data are the clinical data repository, multiple system databases, or stand-alone databases exclusively used for the DSS or ES. These systems cannot aid decision making if they cannot access essential information. Often, due to some of the usability problems discussed regarding CISs, data are incomplete and/or inaccurate, and appropriate decision support cannot be provided. In addition, data accessibility problems can be encountered if the information required for decision support and expert advice resides in many different systems. These data may not be accessible due to technical infrastructure limitations (i.e., incompatible platforms) or nonstandardized data across systems (i.e., data having different meanings in different systems).

Another critical success factor is the validity and ongoing maintenance of the knowledge base (rules and guidelines) by which the system performs analysis and provides recommendations. The primary function of DSSs and ESs is to parse rules and empirical observations to yield valid predictions. Therefore, they must be given current and valid rules and guidelines developed by experts in the relevant fields. If the knowledge base is not correct or up to date, these support systems will make the wrong decisions or recommendations. It is imperative that this component of the system be tested thoroughly and evaluated on an ongoing basis.

Iterative prototyping and ongoing evaluation of the system are also critically important. Iterative prototyping ensures that the end user receives a final product that meets expectations. In the current health care environment, the days of defining requirements and then implementing a system 2 years later are over. This is especially true for DSSs and ESs, whose knowledge bases and uses change almost monthly. Users must be involved in the development process and must provide regular feedback and evaluation following implementation to ensure that the system does not become outdated.[11]

Practice Management Systems

The market for practice management systems (PMSs) has grown with the integration of physicians into delivery organizations. There is a growing recognition that the physician's office is an extension of a larger care delivery process rather than a discrete island of care.[12] With regard to disease management, the PMS allows several key benefits, including

- *Integrated communication with widely dispersed physicians.* The PMS provides the frameworks through which the content of disease management can pass at low marginal costs.
- *Systemwide scheduling and electronic mail–based referrals and replies.* This allows the entity involved in disease management to balance capacity and demand across many disparate sites and permits patients, physicians, or other caregivers to schedule other resources.
- *Centralized (claims) data collection across many practitioners.*
- *Access to laboratory data and other results.* This reduces redundancy and increases throughput of patient care, as well as supporting non–physician-based interventions such as case management.
- *Population research to develop disease-specific interventions.* From the physician database, population data can be assembled and analyzed for corporate disease-specific health services research.

PMSs provide the primary means by which physicians' offices are linked with each other or with a delivery system. They provide an architecture for other systems such as EMRs, DSSs, or ESs to integrate. With a PMS in place, many activities (electronic mail between referring physicians, rapid patient flow across sites of care, or access to laboratory study results performed by other physicians) that enhance the value of disease management can be accomplished.

Community Health Information Networks

Community health information networks (CHINs) began as an effort to bring together the disparate data of a regional population, including that of pharmacies, insurers, employers, hospitals, laboratories, and related agencies. Early efforts envisioned large-scale technical infrastructures and extensive interrelationships for data exchange. However, this vision has generally not been realized for a number of reasons. Primarily, the development of CHINs has been inhibited by the enormous expense of the connectivity infrastructure, the confidentiality and proprietary concerns of the community constituents, the lack of an objective central force or direction, and the conflicting interests of the prospective participants.[13] CHINs' failure to fulfill their promise can also be attributed to a poorly defined constituency, a lack of resolution of competitive issues, conflicts of interest associated with the sharing of proprietary information, unclear expectations of benefits, the lack of technology alignment with business goals, the absence of stepwise implementation, a focus on competitive advantage rather than community advantage, and the nonexistence of internally integrated systems within CHIN members' own organizations.[14]

Although the implementation of CHINs in the traditional sense has met with some difficulty, the concept has heightened recognition of the need for further integrated communities of care. Organizations and groups have formed in many communities to evaluate the health care information needs of their residents and care entities. These groups recognize that at some point the technology costs of linking a community will decrease and that communities must be ready to exchange information for the sake of improved care. Therefore, communities must attempt to overcome nontechnological hurdles, such as competitive barriers to information sharing, to ensure the successful implementation of community health networks. Regardless of the technology used to facilitate the community-wide sharing of information (such as the Internet of the future with expanded bandwidth and capacity), clear benefits can result from this activity.

Two principal areas of progress that have already been recognized by CHINs are master member indexing (MMI) and eligibility maintenance. These processes are illustrated in Figure 5–2. MMI is a response to a simple, pervasive, and unsolved problem. People are given different identification numbers at each institu-

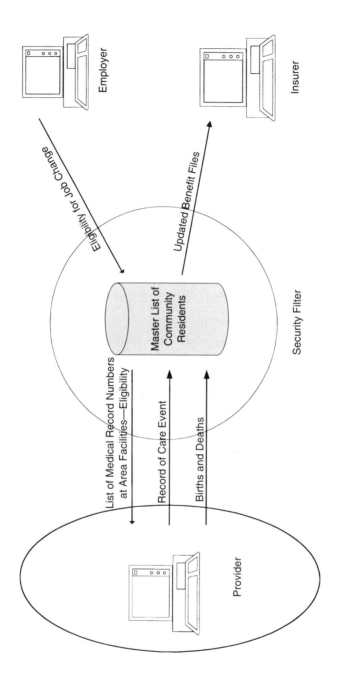

Figure 5–2 Community Health Information Network (CHIN)

tion, pharmacy, physician's office, and other health care sites. There is no way to assemble all of the information relevant to a patient across all of these organizational partitions. An MMI that is well done (multipart codes and not social security numbers) does not put patient confidentiality at risk but can be exceedingly valuable by making test results, drug compliance, symptoms, and utilization data available to any provider or physician. This effort is essential to the success of disease management efforts because of the need to piece together fragments of data to understand and manage disease evolution.

Eligibility maintenance has grown out of the observation that when enrolling new patients, most providers cannot confirm their eligibility. When patients switch health plans, even the health plan cannot identify a specific person as having a particular eligibility. Thus, community and private efforts to assemble current eligibility databases allow more specific treatments, reduce treatment delays, and avoid unnecessary patient copays for therapies outside the eligibility requirements. Eligibility maintenance will be important to disease management as a means of establishing whether patients are treatable in a given disease management program at any time.

In addition, CHINs have the potential to reduce other data and processing duplication activities. Just as the MMI reduces duplication of identification numbers across health care entities, duplicate processes can be eliminated. A physician at a clinic may perform a series of tests or procedures during a patient's visit. When that patient visits a different physician at a local hospital, the same tests or procedures may be performed again due to the lack of information exchange or the unavailability of test results. A CHIN can ensure that the hospital is aware of the tests and procedures that have been performed and that it has access to the associated results.

Further, one of the greatest benefits to disease management is increased population data resources. Since disease management relies on information for disease populations over time, increasing the store of data available increases the prospects of success for disease management. CHINs offer a wider range of available data than that traditionally available to single entities or organizations. Generally, if a hospital wishes to evaluate outcomes for a specific treatment for asthma patients, it is limited to its own data and treatment results. However, with the introduction of other hospitals' experiences provided via a CHIN, the entire community can achieve a more accurate account of its outcomes for specific treatments. In addition, the community can better identify and predict population trends associated with specific diseases.

Though traditional CHINs are expensive and challenging to implement, disease management entities should begin to prepare relationships and resources for an environment of shared community information. As the technology becomes less expensive and more readily available, the competitive basis for healthier organizations will be, not proprietary information, but rather how population information is used to provide higher-quality services at lower costs.

Internet and Intranet Technologies

Internet and Intranet applications have the potential to provide value to all stakeholders in disease management. Providers, physicians, and employers can use Internet and Intranet technologies to obtain easy access to information, practice rules, and performance data. They can also use them to communicate more frequently and conveniently via electronic mail and forums.

These technologies have aided providers and caregivers in communicating with one another more efficiently. In addition, the medical research information and caregiver educational materials available on the Internet have proven to be quite valuable to those provider institutions that have made them easily accessible. Many companies also provide Internet applications and services that allow providers to evaluate their own performance compared to that of others. Providers can use these services to identify trends in care provision and new ways to reduce costs and improve quality. They can also use these services to review member physicians' evaluation scores, make specialist referrals, and process prescription orders for a local pharmacy directly on line.

Employers and other payers for health care service are turning to the Internet as well. Many are offering enrollment and registration services for their various health plans via the Internet. They are also promoting their plans and services via the Internet, allowing potential members to research interactively topics that interest them and ask questions directly on line. Many payer entities are recognizing that they can create new effective ways to reach consumers and influence their purchasing decisions through advanced marketing techniques on the Internet.

The stakeholder who may benefit most from the Internet is the patient, who now has access to a vast array of information sources. If health care delivery organizations can better inform and educate patients, they can tap into one of the primary drivers of health care costs. If patients are more informed, they are likely to seek preventive maintenance more often and live healthier lifestyles. In addition, they are more likely to follow prescribed instructions of caregivers. This will effectively decrease the need for direct patient care and likely improve quality of care and cost effectiveness.

Internet applications currently in production and under development include many educational and informational sources and activities. These applications give patients direct access to information about networks, such as participating physicians and hospitals and types of plans offered. They also can provide the user with access to medical libraries and research articles. Many of the applications include features by which patients can "chat" directly with physicians or nurses, often eliminating the need to visit. Finally, these applications can educate the patient about diseases and how best to live with and treat them. For example, the application may have an Internet page dedicated to living with asthma. The potential benefits and reductions in required care that can result from educated patients are overwhelming. In addition to informing and educating patients, these applications can be used to schedule appointments and order prescriptions.

Since this is a relatively new technology, many health care organizations are unaware of the potential benefits and lack the technical knowledge base necessary to design, develop, and implement an Internet application. However, the technology in and of itself is fairly straightforward. The key is recognizing the benefits it can provide.

Many physicians are concerned that not all of their patients have access to the Internet, and are not sure that those who do have access actually use it for health care information. Currently, it is estimated that only 10% to 20% of the population has regular access to the Internet.[15] Therefore, many patients who could greatly benefit from this type of application cannot use it. The percentage of the population with access continues to increase dramatically, however. Therefore, it is likely that the long-term benefits will be substantial.

DEVELOPMENT AND IMPLEMENTATION

We have explored here how the business plan of entities involved in disease management translates into information systems strategy and how core technologies interrelate to produce information that is valuable in disease management. However, whether driven by the need to manage diseases or by some other core business need, the process of designing, implementing, and using information technology in health care must be approached in a manner that can be successful within a fixed time frame and on a limited budget, while minimizing implementation risks.

The spectrum of risks in implementing disease management information technology ranges from moving too ambitiously in systems implementation to moving too slowly so that the market shift that creates the opportunity closes without exploitation. Either manifestation can lead to permanent loss of disease management market opportunities. Though risks cannot be completely mitigated, an implementation methodology is needed that translates the business strategy into a technology plan and at the same time breaks this plan into manageable steps. In this way, market opportunities can be exploited without leading to actual or perceived failure of product delivery.

Numerous technology implementation methods have been described that are generally useful to disease management information systems. These methods fall largely into two major categories. First are those governing technology changes that are not accompanied by changes in the general business plan of the organization, such as the replacement of transaction systems with clinical information systems or the displacement of computed tomography (CT) scanners by magnetic resonance imaging (MRIs). Second are those governing technology changes that result from shifts in the business strategy of the organization (largely due to market shifts). In this case, because the business strategy itself has changed, old information systems may slow the evolution of the new business model, while at the same time desired technology may not be feasible or available.

Planning and implementing disease management technology requires combining new technologies and new business strategies. It involves paying attention to both the technology changes and the business model changes to which they are applied. Disease management represents a substantial shift in the business strategy of providers, suppliers, and physicians and a different level of engagement for employers and patients. At the same time, the information technology support underlying disease management is new to the health care market in many ways. It is clinical, distributed on a large scale, directly used by caregivers and other stakeholders, longitudinal, and "real time." To a considerable degree, the advent of modern technology has permitted disease management, unlike many other patient care approaches, actually to fulfill the hopes held for it. The following sections briefly review key issues involved in implementing technology for disease management.

Business Strategy

Although it may seem unlikely, the key source of success in technology implementation is the business plan. As an expensive capital investment, information systems require a business framework that defines what to expect from the technology, over what time frame the technology must perform, and how the benefits of the technology should be measured. In many cases, unsuccessful information systems implementation can be directly attributed to a lack of a clear business strategy.

Implementation of information systems for disease management requires a disciplined assessment of which stakeholders are being served by the initiative, which business steps are being performed by the entity involved in disease management, and which benefits will be delivered to the stakeholders. Given the broad and possibly conflicting needs of stakeholders, the business plan must narrow the focus if the technology implementation is to be affordable and feasible.

Because many disease management ventures are offering new services and interventions that have not been available, many of the functions required must be created *de novo*. This further implies that the information system technology needed to perform them probably can be neither bought "off the shelf" nor modified from existing systems. Therefore, the business plan must demonstrate how it will enhance the service and information offering of the entity so that relevant information technology can be implemented in phases.

The business plan must address the capital required to implement information technology. The capital plan should cover the hardware, the software and operating system, applications, telecommunications, and maintenance/operations. The business plan should describe the role of the core technologies, how they will interrelate, and how they will be modified and enhanced to support fully the information needs of disease management.

Technology Master Plan

The stakeholder needs identified in the completed business plan must be translated into a technology master plan outlining the architecture of the technologies, the scope of requirements needed to provide minimal functionality, and the timetable of deliverables that can support the business entity. The technology master plan should also detail the acquisition plan of specific hardware, applications, and peripherals and how the sequencing of these investments will be managed.

The master plan is more than a "materials and scope of function" plan. It should detail what functionality is required in the system, how the design process will be managed, and how user acceptance and training will be accomplished. The design process should be one that outlines the source of user/customer inputs, how proof of concept and prototyping will be handled, and how the release cycle will be managed (e.g., how often modified versions of software will be released and controlled). The master plan will set forth the roles of users in testing and how end users will be trained and maintained.

The business plan and the technology master plan set the framework for how business needs and technology capabilities interdependently shape the role of information systems. However, the constraint imposed by the market's narrow window of opportunity for successful deployment of disease management systems is a nontechnological constraint with significant technology implications. Simply put, the entity must deliver services and information within a time horizon shorter than that in which the technology can be adopted and successfully deployed. Indeed, without the near-term success of basic information system functionality, the entity involved in disease management will fail. Likewise, without technology implementation in the presence of a well-considered plan, the entity will also fail. This implies (1) that a combination of long-range planning and short-run implementation is required to be successful in the disease management market and (2) that incremental or stepwise implementation methods must be a prominent feature of disease management technology planning.

The business plan and the technology plan should state how a return on investment (e.g., measurable qualitative and quantitative benefits that outweigh the associated costs) will result from the technology implementation. Although the returns from a technology investment do not necessarily have to yield financial benefits, justifying technology investments on the basis of "strategic necessity" (e.g., an often unjustified claim that an investment is necessary for "strategic" reasons without demonstrated return on investment or support for the business plan) should be avoided.

Design and Implementation

Whether an organization is developing information systems in house or is outsourcing the development effort, a number of steps help ensure a successful end product. The following list identifies and briefly discusses an important subset of practices that are most commonly neglected:

1. *Maintain active communication.* Listen to and read about stakeholders, and talk to and write to them. Educate stakeholders about what they should expect, and encourage them to tell developers what they want.
2. *Define the objectives.* State clearly what the purpose and role of the system will be and how the system will affect the work of those involved.
3. *Obtain support from key individuals or groups.* Get support for the system from key individuals and their constituencies, including end users, those with authority over the project, those with financial control of the project, informal leaders whose opinions are respected and sought, and those with the skills and knowledge base necessary to implement the technology.
4. *Involve users from start to finish.* Involve a subset of those users in the requirements definition for the system, design of the system, testing of the system, and postimplementation evaluation of the system.
5. *Identify critical success factors early.* Identify any factor that will cause the systems effort to fail, and make contingency plans.
6. *Plan for administration, maintenance, and user support.* Plan for the increased overhead—both financial and human resource—for system administration, maintenance, and user support functions.
7. *Plan for conversion and systems integration.* Start planning for conversion and integration with other systems early in the development process so that data contents selected for the new system are compatible with the needs of other systems.

Selecting Vendors and Products

Although some health care organizations possess the resources to design, develop, and implement new systems successfully, many must rely on third-party products and vendors to meet their needs. Thoroughly evaluating and selecting a third-party vendor and product can be resource intensive, but its benefits greatly justify its costs. Health care organizations regularly experience frustration with products that do not support their requirements or with vendors that do not perform as promised. However, there are many excellent products and responsible vendors committed to service and excellence. The task for the disease management entity in selecting a software product and vendor is to determine which vendors and products have strengths where they are necessary and which vendor or product weaknesses are inconsequential.

Once the business and systems objectives have been defined, the entity must develop or have access to the relevant technical and functional skills and knowledge to evaluate intelligently its vendors and products. Next, a broad list of products and vendors that meet the requirements should be developed. This can be accomplished by reviewing health care information technology surveys and magazines, researching the topic on the Internet, networking with other entities to determine what products they use, or seeking the support of a consulting or research services firm. Once the group of contending vendors and products has been established, a set of evaluation criteria should be designed, and each alternative should be evaluated based on these criteria. It is helpful to evaluate first the alternatives on only a subset of the most important criteria to narrow the options for a more detailed analysis.

Although the criteria employed to evaluate a vendor differ among organizations, some common factors are often used. When developing criteria on which to evaluate a product vendor, some of the following questions may be useful:

1. *Longevity.* How long has the vendor been in the business of providing products similar to the one that must be procured? Is the vendor's profitability and long-term business outlook positive?
2. *Product support.* Does this vendor offer after-purchase support? If so, how expensive is it, and what type of support is it?
3. *Reputation and recommendations.* Does this vendor have a good reputation for producing excellent products and providing outstanding service? What are the opinions of organizations that have previously dealt with this vendor?
4. *Product line offering.* Is this the only product in which the vendor has production experience? What other related products does the vendor offer?

There are also a variety of criteria for evaluating software products. The list below identifies some of the most important and commonly asked questions.

1. *Requirements support.* Does the product meet the business and system requirements? Does it have the documentation necessary to determine if it meets the requirements?

2. *Platform and environment compatibility.* Will the product operate correctly on an organization's technical platform and in an organization's technical environment?

3. *Open orientation and expandability.* Can this product communicate and exchange data with other products without a great deal of modification and expended resources? Can this product be easily expanded to support a broader range of functions?

4. *Usability and flexibility.* Can the organization's users use the product in their day-to-day environment? Is the product's interface intuitive or more likely to cause data entry problems and misinterpretation? Can the product be configured to meet the unique needs of different users?

5. *Product track record.* How long has this product been in use? What do previous users have to say about it? Is the product fully developed, or is it a demonstration?

6. *On-line help and support.* Does the product provide sufficient on-line help and support for users to answer real-time questions?

7. *Training requirements and support.* Does the vendor provide product training? If so, how expensive is that training? If not, how difficult is it to train new users on the system? Is the system intuitive enough so that it does not require an extraordinary amount of training?

8. *Warranty.* Who pays for problems with the software? Who must correct the problem, and how long should it take to correct the problem? What is covered under the warranty, and for how long?

If these considerations are addressed in the evaluation of the product alternatives, most of the major problems that often plague organizations during the after-purchase phase can be minimized. Table 5–3 summarizes evaluation criteria for both vendors and products.

DISCUSSION AND CONCLUSIONS

This chapter has examined the way information technology affects the success and failure of disease management programs. There are several caveats for those who are implementing disease management initiatives. First, disease management is a business strategy that has broad interpretation to many stakeholders in the delivery system. Therefore, few prescriptions can be offered about the information systems requirements. Second, the role that each stakeholder plays in disease management is different. Hence, the way each invests in information technology, and how each should judge the costs and benefits of that investment, will vary. Moreover, those who try to satisfy the needs of multiple stakeholders may not see synergy between investments made to satisfy each. Third, it is difficult to separate

Table 5–3 Evaluation Criteria for Vendors and Products

Vendor	Product
Longevity	Requirements support
Product support	Platform and environment compatibility
Reputation and recommendations	Open orientation and expandability
Product line offering	Usability and flexibility
	Product track record
	On-line help and support
	Training requirements and support
	Warranty

the specific business strategy of disease management from overall market trends. Therefore, it is also difficult to articulate a disease management information systems strategy that is separable from the general life cycle of technology needed to operate any health care organization. Fourth, rapidly evolving changes in the technology markets make it difficult to identify the specific technologies that are "best" for disease management for a horizon longer than several months. Finally, there is a conflict between the imperative to take bold steps in order to take advantage of opportunities presented by the disease management market and the cautious, careful nature of information systems development that leads to successfully deployed technology.

Despite these cautions, a few clear strategies emerge for using information technology in disease management. First, information technology can be used to create a common view of a disease across stakeholders by use of education and communication. This commonality is critical for all stakeholders to manage disease with common goals and for hand-off problems between stakeholders to be reduced. Second, information technology can be used to improve the effectiveness and efficiency of disease prevention and treatment. In the end, the ability to prevent disease and to treat safely and effectively is the overarching common goal of disease management and, indeed, of medicine. Information technology can improve physician performance, provider management, and the role of employers and patients. Third, information technology can enhance the role of the patient. All stakeholders will be able to manage diseases better if patients become more empowered, discriminating, and active in their care. Fourth, information technology can measure the value of alternatives in health care. For years, the test in health care has been "Does this test or therapy add benefit?" With its focus on using limited resources wisely, disease management asks, "What is the most effective and efficient way to treat or prevent disease?" The demonstration of this value will enhance the ability of all stakeholders to manage and reduce the burden of disease. In this way, disease management may fulfill the high expectations we place on it.

References

1. Pauly MV. *Doctors and Their Workshops*. Chicago, Ill: University of Chicago Press; 1980.
2. Wyatt CJ. Clinical data systems, part 1: data and medical records. *Lancet*. 1994;344:1543–1547.
3. Wyatt CJ. Clinical data systems, part 3: development and evaluation. *Lancet*. 1994;344:1682–1688.
4. Tan JT, Hanna J. Integrating health care with information technology: knitting patient information through networking. *Health Care Manage Rev*. 1994;19(2):72–80.
5. Morrissey J. Interface engines rev up. *Mod Health Care*. 1995;25(19):49–60.
6. Branger PJ, van der Wouden JC, Schudel BR, et al. Electronic communication between providers of primary and secondary care. *Br Med J*. 1992;305:1068–1070.
7. Schaich RL. Making the case for EDI. *Comput Health Care*. 1993;14(3):18–22.
8. Andrew WF, Dick RS. Applied information technology: a clinical perspective feature focus: the computer-based patient record (part 2). *Comput Nurs*. 1995;13(3):80–84.
9. Amataykul M. CPR definition becoming clearer. *Health Manage Technol*. 1995;16(8):66–76.
10. Keegan AJ, Baldwin B. EIS: a better way to view hospital trends. *Health Care Finan Manage*. 1992;46(11):58–66.
11. Wyatt J, Spiegelhalter D. Evaluating medical expert systems: what to test and how? *Med Inf*. 1990;15(3):205–217.
12. Edelson JT. Physician use of information technology in ambulatory medicine: an overview. *J Ambul Care Manage*. 1995;18(3):9–17.
13. Appleby C. The trouble with CHINs. *Hosp Health Networks*. 1995;69(9):42–44.
14. Work M, Pawola L. CHINs, IHD systems remain in evolutionary state. *Health Manage Technol*. 1996;17(3):54–58.
15. Braly D. Enterprise-wide scheduling: do you need it? *Health Manage Technol*. 1996;17(6):32.

CHAPTER 6

Disease Management: Making It Work—A Study in Implementation Strategies and Results in an Integrated Delivery System

John J. Byrnes, John Lucas, and Margaret J. Gunter

In a recent editorial, Dr. David Nash from Thomas Jefferson University stated:

> The proliferation of disease management programs, practice guidelines, and case management teams makes one think that all managed care organizations and integrated delivery systems are making great strides in the care of patients with chronic illnesses. Yet, in a search of the published literature, very little progress is discernible and, to my chagrin, more heat than light appears to have been generated.[1]

Indeed, many well-respected health care organizations had been successful in developing guidelines, protocols, and narrowly focused disease management interventions. But few have demonstrated successful implementation of such programs, particularly across an entire continuum of care for a given disease.

One recent successful program discussed by Nash, as well as by Gunter et al,[2] has been instituted by Lovelace Health Systems, an integrated delivery system located in Albuquerque, New Mexico. Entitled EPISODES OF CARE™ (EOC™), it is a disease management program that continues to demonstrate substantial improvements in patient treatment across a variety of chronic, complex diseases. Case examples from this program are the subject of this chapter. Reviews will be provided of interventions for depression, diabetes, birth, prematurity prevention, and pediatric asthma, focusing on successful implementation strategies and lessons learned.

LOVELACE HEALTH SYSTEMS

Lovelace Health Systems is the largest and most fully integrated health care system in New Mexico. In addition to 320 staff-model physicians, the system includes a 235-bed hospital, a behavioral health care center, nine primary care centers in Albuquerque, four regional practice sites, a 1600-physician IPA, six affiliated research institutes, and a health plan with over 160,000 members, representing over 40% of the market.

The Albuquerque marketplace is characterized as highly integrated, with approximately 70% penetration by managed care. It is identified, along with areas such as Minneapolis and various California regions, as one of the most advanced markets in the country. The need to remain competitive in this area of intense competition was a major impetus to the creation of the Lovelace EPISODES OF CARE™ program and related population health management strategies.[3]

EPISODES OF CARE™

The goal of the EPISODES OF CARE™ program is to reengineer patient care across the entire continuum for given disease states. From inpatient and outpatient databases, diseases are selected that are of the highest volume and cost to the system, thus allowing strategic targeting of scarce internal resources for quality improvement. The program is also founded on the principle that cost follows quality—that as improvements in quality are made, efficiency and cost reductions automatically follow. In the majority of cases in the EOC™ program, this has proven true.

Birth EPISODES OF CARE™

Long before the subject of Caesarean section (hereafter "C-section") rates became a national issue, the physicians and midwives within Lovelace Health Systems identified this area for a focused improvement effort. As illustrated in Figure 6–1, the C-section rate in 1989 was 23%, a respectable level for that year. The rate is now 13% for 1996, well below the U.S. Public Health Service goal for the year 2000.

When asked to outline the interventions that made the improvements in C-section rates possible, Dr. Shelburne, Chairman of OB/GYN, provided this list:

1. the practice philosophy of the midwives
2. the review of each C-section by department members
3. a multidisciplinary (24 hour) in-house team made up of physicians and midwives

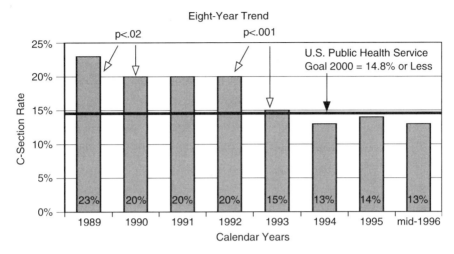

Figure 6–1 Lovelace Hospital C-Section Rate Changes. Courtesy of Lovelace Healthcare Innovations and Lovelace Health Systems, Albuquerque, New Mexico.

---

4. standardization of practice protocols and guidelines
5. a highly developed set of nursing protocols

What was particularly noteworthy was the group's ability to maintain the improvements from year to year. This trend demonstrated the integration of practice improvement protocols into the fabric of daily medical practice. In other words, the group was able to make fundamental changes at a very practical level in the way they delivered care to their patients. These changes were incorporated into the tools, standard orders, and policies and procedures that provide the operational foundation for the department.

This case also demonstrates the optimal quality of care that can be obtained when providers use a synergistic (integrated) team approach to care delivery. The union of the midwives' philosophy with that of the physicians and the labor and delivery (L&D) nurses had a profound impact on the quality of care and service delivered to patients. The review of each C-section during department meetings provided a powerful forum for discussion and learning. Building upon the concept of the small learning group, this practice provided a safe educational venue when used in the spirit of mutual understanding. It provided a mechanism for shared learning, reinforcement of practice guidelines, and an opportunity for collegial discussion and exchange. When it was conducted with all provider groups in attendance, team spirit, understanding, and trust were likewise improved.

The use of a 24-hour in-house team removed many of the subtle and often sub-conscious elements that influence medical decision making. The team was in house, immediately available to handle questions, consultations, or emergencies in person. There was no hurry to complete deliveries before dinnertime or before colleagues assumed care responsibilities in the morning.

Standardization of practice protocols and guidelines, when incorporated as a fundamental working of the practice, removed much of the provider-to-provider practice variation. The indications for C-section became well known to all team members, practice became more uniform, and improvements in outcomes were self-evident.

Depression EPISODES OF CARE™

The depression EOC™ was chartered with the realization that depression was probably underdiagnosed and undertreated within the Lovelace system. Current literature tells us that this situation is common within the American health system. With the advent of more effective treatments, it was considered prudent to im-prove practice for this chronic, complex condition.

In 1993, a multidisciplinary team was assembled to examine and redesign the entire continuum of care for depression. As one of the original nine EOC™ teams, the depression team met the criteria for selection due to the disorder's (1) high volume of patients, (2) high cost of underdiagnosis, (3) high risk to the patient if undiagnosed, and (4) tremendous opportunity for improvement in care.

The depression EOC™ team was led by two co-champions: a psychiatrist and a family practice physician. Other members of the team included quality department staff, other physicians, nurses, care managers, social workers, and an administra-tor. This model was used throughout the EOC™ program. It has been Lovelace's experience that physician-directed teams have been instrumental to the EOC™ program success. Likewise, the pairing of specialist and primary care physicians as cochampions facilitated the buy-in of both stakeholder groups and a spirit of collegiality.

The depression EOC™ team set out to accomplish the following:

1. *Engage the primary care physicians* and mental health providers in a team approach to improving the quality of care for depressed patients
2. *Increase awareness* among all providers of the incidence of depression in their practices
3. *Increase the comfort* of primary care physicians in treating depression within the primary care setting

To accomplish these goals, the team developed a series of interventions. First, provider-friendly practice guidelines were developed. Using guidelines readily available from the public domain, the team customized the guidelines to the Lovelace environment.

A key design feature for practice guidelines incorporated the "Greenberg rule," in honor of the primary care co-champion of this team. The Greenberg rule states, "A useful practice guideline must be distilled into one page." This one page contains the most important aspects of the guideline and the targets for improvement. This first page is supported by detailed guidelines and treatment recommendations readily available to providers. This key design element is now incorporated into all EOC™ practice guidelines.

The team also focused on locating a practice support tool that would enable providers to diagnose depression more easily and more objectively. Several instruments were evaluated, and the Zung scale was ultimately selected (see Exhibit 6–1). Initially, adoption by the primary care providers was not as successful as envisioned. To demonstrate the utility of this tool, the author made an adjustment to the provider education program. Rather than simply talking about or showing the tool during continuing medical education (CME) training, educators distributed the Zung scale to the audience and had the audience fill it out themselves. Once hesitancy and skepticism were overcome, this exercise proved very successful in demonstrating the utility of the instrument at a very practical level. Use of the scale subsequently increased nicely (see Figure 6–2).

On the education front, focus groups with Lovelace primary care physicians made it clear that they preferred education programs to be short, highly focused, very practical, and immediately useful. Hence, CME training was limited to 45 minutes in duration and focused on the tools to support the physicians. Physicians also wanted to be taught by a practicing peer whom they respected and who had incorporated the EOC™ system into his or her own practice. This strategy has proven very successful. Dr. Greenberg is now the internal champion for the depression project and states that "it has been one of the most fulfilling experiences in my medical career."

The behavioral specialists also wanted to support fully their primary care colleagues by making telephone consultation immediately available. In this way, guidance could be provided to primary care physicians while patients were still in their offices. This provided several advantages to all parties. The patient was often spared a formal referral and an additional visit with another provider. The primary care physician could more immediately meet patients' needs. A treatment plan was developed and implemented before the patient left the office. This takes advantage of the "teachable moment" between primary care physician (PCP) and

Exhibit 6–1 Zung Scale for Depression

Instructions: Read each sentence carefully. For each statement, check the bubble that best corresponds to how often you have felt that way during the past two weeks. Please check a response for each of the 23 items.
   * For statements 5 and 7, if you are on a diet, answer as if you were not.

	None or a little of the time	Some of the time	Good part of the time	Most or all of the time
1. I feel downhearted, blue, and sad.	○	○	○	○
2. Morning is when I feel the best.	○	○	○	○
3. I have crying spells or feel like it.	○	○	○	○
4. I have trouble sleeping through the night.	○	○	○	○
5. I eat as much as I used to.*	○	○	○	○
6. I enjoy looking at, talking to, and being with attractive women/men.	○	○	○	○
7. I notice that I am losing weight.*	○	○	○	○
8. I have trouble with constipation.	○	○	○	○
9. My heart beats faster than usual.	○	○	○	○
10. I get tired for no reason.	○	○	○	○
11. My mind is as clear as it used to be.	○	○	○	○
12. I find it easy to do the things I used to do.	○	○	○	○
13. I am restless and can't keep still.	○	○	○	○
14. I feel hopeful about the future.	○	○	○	○
15. I am more irritable than usual.	○	○	○	○
16. I find it easy to make decisions.	○	○	○	○
17. I feel that I am useful and needed.	○	○	○	○
18. My life is pretty full.	○	○	○	○
19. I feel that others would be better off if I were dead.	○	○	○	○
20. I still enjoy the things I used to do.	○	○	○	○
21. Are you currently taking medication for depression?	○ yes	○ no		
22. Are you currently in counseling for depression?	○ yes	○ no		
23. Have you ever been diagnosed with depression?	○ yes	○ no		

Source: Copyright © Elizabeth Zung

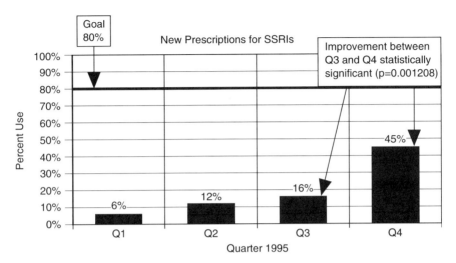

Figure 6–2 Percentage of Zung Scale Use. Courtesy of Lovelace Healthcare Innovations and Lovelace Health Systems, Albuquerque, New Mexico.

specialist physicians, one of the most powerful adult teaching tools available. Finally, the immediate availability of specialists created a sense of collegiality and partnership among the providers. The behavioral care hotline was fondly called "1-800-dial-a-shrink," the name coined by the chair of behavioral health.

Diabetes EPISODES OF CARE™

The diabetes EOC™ was chartered because of diabetes' position as one of the top-ranking diagnoses based on volume and cost data (for both inpatients and outpatients) within Lovelace Health Systems. New Mexico also has the distinction of serving a population that has twice the national incidence of diabetes.

Drawing upon the expertise of a long-standing American Diabetes Association–approved program and a dedicated group of providers, certified diabetes educators, and nurses, the EOC™ team sought to

1. improve process indicators for acute management of diabetes
2. improve outcome indicators for chronic management of diabetes as related to long-term complications
3. demonstrate benchmark-level performance for retinal eye exam rates
4. provide useful practice support tools for providers throughout the system, including electronic and practice profiling strategies

5. better engage patients in the management of their disease
6. integrate the depression EOC™ into the diabetes EOC™ due to the high incidence of depression in the diabetic population[3]

The diabetes team developed a number of innovative provider support tools that won immediate endorsement from providers throughout the system. The first was a patient-specific report that was integrated into the electronic medical record (see Exhibit 6–2). This report contained several important elements required for successful disease management implementation. First, useful, practical, patient-specific data were made immediately available at the time of the patient visit to support clinical decision making. Second, the report listed the quality indicators targeted for improvement and tracked them for all diabetic patients within the system:

- glycosylated hemoglobin levels
- microalbumin
- date of patient education
- date of patient retinal exam
- other laboratory results

Exhibit 6–2 Diabetes Patient-Specific Electronic Report

Profile Screen—Electronic
Diabetes Care—Treatment Summary

	Glyco-hemoglobin	Micro-albumin	Ret. Exam	Educ.	Chol.	HDL	LDL	TRIG
Due						X	X	X
7/13/95	9.6 Min.	32 High			150			
1/23/95	9.4 Int.				185			
8/24/94				X				
9/14/93			X					

Remember Foot Exam
If Microalbumin is High Consider ACE!
30% of patients with diabetes may be depressed—
administer Zung scale

Courtesy of Lovelace Healthcare Innovations and Lovelace Health Systems, Albuquerque, New Mexico.

Third, the top line of the report indicated the test(s) or intervention(s) due at the time of the clinic visit. Fourth, several key leverage points within the practice guideline were listed as reminders for the provider.

The report makes a provider's practice more efficient by eliminating the drudgery of looking through paper records, trying to locate missing records, or placing multiple calls to locate reports. This illustrates a cardinal tenet: all disease management interventions, designs, and systems must make a provider's job easier, more efficient, and more effective. Interventions that add work or prolong patient visits are never implemented.

Two additional screens follow that provide an overview of the practice guideline (Exhibit 6–3) with suggestions for steps involved in a focused diabetic visit (Exhibit 6–4). The screens are immediately available to support a provider at the time of visit.

The second provider support tool is the Provider Support Report (see Exhibit 6–5). It profiles a provider's practice in a number of ways. First, all diabetic patients within the provider's practice are queried. Each patient is compared against the indicators tracked and identified as being within or outside the standard. The provider's performance is then scored against these standards, as illustrated in the upper left-hand corner. In this instance, 78% of Dr. Cure's diabetic patients had retinal eye exams completed within the recommended interval.

Next, Dr. Cure's performance is compared to her practice location as well as to her entire peer group of primary care providers in the Lovelace system. This is illustrated in the upper right-hand corner of the report. This provides Dr. Cure with comparisons she can use for benchmarking her performance relative to that of her colleagues.

The most powerful part of the report is located at the bottom. It provides a listing of each patient within Dr. Cure's practice who falls outside the standard and on which indicators. With this information, Dr. Cure or her office staff can call the listed patients and schedule the appropriate appointment. Improvements can be dramatic.

To obtain this level of detail in the past, Dr. Cure would have needed to perform a comprehensive chart review on each diabetic patient in her practice every quarter. Therein lies the power of this report. It is produced quarterly by the EOC™ department as a service to Lovelace physicians. The data elements are obtained from standard health system databases—claims, pharmacy, and laboratory.

Finally, this report is used for practice support and education only. In the spirit of collegiality and partnership with the physicians, it provides a means to deliver optimal care to patients. Within the Lovelace organization, profiling information of this type is not used in a punitive manner or for "bad apple" hunting. Thus, it becomes not a tool to be feared but one that is requested and immediately useful.

With these and a number of other strategies in progress, particularly intense patient education and treatment of concomitant depression, Lovelace has started

Exhibit 6–3 The Focused Diabetes Visit, Overview Screen

The Focused Diabetes Visit

Diet   Complications Screening
Insulin/Oral Agents   Reactions/Hypoglycemia
Exercise/Education   Assess Attitude/Barriers to Care
Testing/Evaluation of Glucose Control   Plan

Blood Glucose Control	*Acceptable*	*Tight*
Fasting serum glucose	70–140 mg/dl	70–120 mg/dl
2 hour post prandial	<200 mg/dl	<160 mg/dl
Glycohemoglobin (5–8.2%)	<10.5%	<9.5%

Complication Screening

Retinopathy: Annual dilated eye exam
Nephropathy: Microalbumin/creatinine ratio annually (first a.m. urine
                    preferred)
                 Normal   <30 mcg/mg creatinine
                 Microalbumin   30–300 mcg/mg creatinine
                 Macroalbumin   >300 mcg/mg creatinine

Lipids (LDL Goals): If no CAD <130, if CAD present <100
Start medication if LDL >160, or if CAD is present and LDL >130 (after diet
    intervention)
Consider medication (gemfibrozil) for TRIG >200 and LDL/HDL >5

Blood pressure should be maintained <130/86
Patients with DM should be considered to have 2 CV risk factors and follow
    Lovelace Lipid Management guidelines

Courtesy of Lovelace Healthcare Innovations and Lovelace Health Systems, Albuquerque,
New Mexico.

---

to see significant improvements in the percentage of patients in good to optimal control of their diabetes (see Figure 6–3). Lovelace hopes to see this rate continue to rise as both reports achieve widespread use.

Prematurity Prevention Program (PPP)

Of the many disease management initiatives in progress, those to reduce the incidence of low–birth weight babies and preterm deliveries are two of the most important. Nationally, the preterm delivery rate is 10.6%, and for New Mexico it

Exhibit 6–4 The Focused Diabetes Visit: Close-up Screen

The Focused Diabetes Visit

Diet   Complications Screening

Insulin/Oral Agents   Reactions/Hypoglycemia

Exercise/Education   Assess Attitude/Barriers to Care

Testing/Evaluation of   Plan

Glucose Control

Courtesy of Lovelace Healthcare Innovations and Lovelace Health Systems, Albuquerque, New Mexico.

is 7.7%. National low–birth weight rates (<2500 g) and very low–birth weight rates (<1500 g) run at 7.1% and 1.3%, respectively. This represents a tremendous opportunity for improvement. As Lovelace has demonstrated, highly focused interventions can dramatically reduce these rates in a very short time.

In an article that appeared in the New Mexico press,[4] Dr. Dale Alverson, Director of Neonatology at the University of New Mexico, stated, "What is incredibly profound was that the number of Lovelace babies in the NICU [neonatal intensive care unit] decreased so dramatically." He was referring to the dramatic change that occurred between 1993 and 1994 after full implementation of the Lovelace Prematurity Prevention Program (PPP). In 1993, the number of NICU admissions totaled 84. In 1994, that number had dropped to 37 while the number of total deliveries (approximately 2000) and patient demographics remained the same. Additionally, the PPP reduced the number of NICU hospital days by 59% and the incidence of preterm deliveries due solely to preterm labor by 38%. Refer to Figures 6–4 and 6–5 for illustrations of further trends in Lovelace in low–birth weight and very low–birth weight deliveries for the 1994–1995 time period.

The accomplishments of the PPP team demonstrated the effectiveness of an aggressive care management (telemanagement) program. Although there were many models for care management, the PPP program relied on an efficient, straightforward approach to implementation, including the following:

1. Early identification and ease of access to prenatal care were stressed. Lovelace achieved a 91% first-trimester prenatal visit rate for 1995. Lovelace waived all copays for prenatal care.
2. All patients were screened for risk of preterm delivery. Patients identified as being at risk were referred into the PPP program.

Exhibit 6-5 The Provider Support Report

Susan Cure

Criteria	Standards	Total Pts w/ Diabetes	Total Pts Tested	# Within Standard	% Within Standard
Education	Rolling 2 yr	35	11	5	45%
Eye Exam	Rolling 1 yr	35	11	8	73%
Foot Exams		35	5	5	100%
Glipizide	<20 mg/day	25	4	4	100%
Glyburide	<15 mg/day	25	0	0	NA
GlycoHb Level	<10.5 mg/day	20	17	2	12%
GlycoHb Ordered	Within 1 yr				
Micro-albumin Ordered	Within 1 yr				
Test Strips					

Percentage of Patients within Standard   01/01/96

■ Provider   ■ Location   □ Primary Care

Patients Outside of Standards

Name	MRN	Pt Ed	Eye Exams	Foot Exams	Glipizide	Glyburide	GlycoHb Level	GlycoHb Ordered	Mircoalbumin	Test Strips
John Doe	XXXXXXXX	N								
Jane Doe	XXXXXXXX						21.40			
Juan Diaz	XXXXXXXX	N					11.90			
Maria Diaz	XXXXXXXX						14.60			

Courtesy of Lovelace Healthcare Innovations and Lovelace Health Systems, Albuquerque, New Mexico.

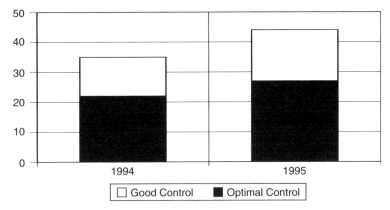

Figure 6–3 Glycemic Control (Glycohemoglobin) among Diabetes Patients. Courtesy of Lovelace Healthcare Innovations and Lovelace Health Systems, Albuquerque, New Mexico.

3. Once enrolled in the PPP program, patients met with the care manager and also received a series of educational materials and interventions appropriate to their condition.
4. Patients were then contacted (at a *minimum*) weekly by the nurse care manager to check status and reinforce education. Patients also received phone numbers for immediate access to caregivers within the Lovelace system.
5. If preterm labor or any signs of increased risk developed, patients were immediately triaged to the appropriate provider for acute treatment.

Simply stated, a coordinated care management program, in cooperation with providers using a multidisciplinary team approach, was a very effective strategy for improving the delivery of care. It represented better care and better outcomes at a more affordable price.[5,6]

The underlying strategy is that the provider group takes a proactive role in managing the health of patients. This is a significant change from the way that traditional health care systems and providers did business. Traditional medical care is and has long been delivered on an "as-needed" basis in a reactive model. Little prevention or proactive care takes place. In facility settings, the quality of care is lower and the cost much higher because when the patients do present to facilities, they are sicker, and the interventions required are more costly.

It is our firm belief that providers of the future will use many proactive systems to deliver care. Because of the results of the PPP program, several telemanagement programs are being implemented within Lovelace Health Systems. Areas of current focus include congestive heart failure, postcardiac bypass (acute phase, when readmissions are common), asthma, and depression.

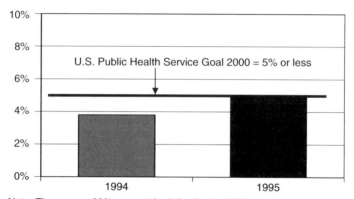

Note: There were 60% more twin deliveries in 1995 compared to 1994, and there was one set of triplets in 1995.

Figure 6–4 Low–Birth Weight Deliveries at Lovelace in 1994 and 1995 (HEDIS Report). Courtesy of Lovelace Healthcare Innovations and Lovelace Health Systems, Albuquerque, New Mexico.

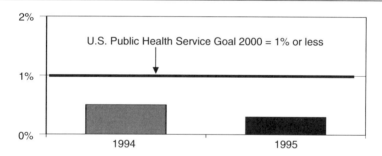

Figure 6–5 Very Low–Birth Weight Deliveries at Lovelace in 1994 and 1995 (HEDIS Report). Courtesy of Lovelace Healthcare Innovations and Lovelace Health Systems, Albuquerque, New Mexico.

Pediatric Asthma EPISODES OF CARE™

The pediatric asthma EOC™ has been a goldmine of lessons learned and pitfalls to avoid. Several years in the making, this platform has been plagued by a variety of obstacles, including turf wars among physicians, nonparticipation by the pediatrics department, and low levels of implementation within family practice. The origin of many of these barriers has been traced to the composition of membership on the EOC™ team. As this has been corrected, implementation has improved significantly.

All EOC™ teams are multidisciplinary in design and are led by team co-champions: a primary care physician and a specialist. The purpose of this design is to nurture collegiality among and between primary care and the various specialty departments. It is also designed to prevent specialty care from directing primary care protocols and designs without significant input from the end users.

Selection of the team co-champions is critical. Most team failures observed within Lovelace have resulted from less-than-optimal selection of team leaders. The leader's ability to build relationships with constituencies, persuade colleagues to try something new, and to mediate, negotiate, and resolve conflicts is paramount. The team leaders need to forge strong bonds and relationships with many different interest groups by invoking the shared purpose of providing optimal patient care. This requires the selection of very special individuals for this leadership role.

The pediatric asthma EOC™ team has also demonstrated a significant design template now being emulated by at least one other EOC™ team. In the beginning, one of the goals of the EOC™ program was to move as much care as appropriate into the primary care arena. Thus, most of the designs were focused upon primary care physicians as the end users, often the only end users. However, the pediatric asthma EOC™ team took a two-pronged approach: (1) the design of protocols was for use in the primary care setting, and (2) the establishment of a Pediatric Asthma Clinic (PAC) was for the purpose of intense education of pediatric patients and their caregivers. Originally staffed only by specialists, the clinic is enjoying an increase in use since a family practice physician has been added to the staff.

The clinic serves as a one-stop educational experience for the patient. Patients are referred by their primary care physician or by automatic referral after a hospitalization. Once the patient and caregiver have completed the educational curriculum, they are referred back to the referring physician for continued care. In this way, the clinic operates as a service to the referring physicians, most of whom are primary care. This guarantee of return of the patient to the referring physician has been critical to the program's success.

The patient- and provider-directed goals of the pediatric asthma EOC™ were to

1. provide a service that delivered one-stop shopping for all asthma needs
2. assist primary care physicians in managing their patients
3. provide a resource for provider, patient, and caregiver education
4. centralize care management and follow-up of high-risk patients
5. facilitate primary care and specialist interaction
6. reduce the need for acute rescue interventions
7. reduce the incidence of hospital admissions and emergency department visits
8. improve the appropriateness of pharmaceutical use specifically related to inhaled steroid and bronchodilators
9. decrease days lost from work by the caregiver, and decrease days lost from school by the patient

10. improve the severity rating for the population of pediatric patients
11. improve patient satisfaction significantly

The illustrations that follow (Figures 6–6 through 6–13) show that this program has enjoyed phenomenal success in delivering optimal care to the pediatric patients. This EOC™ demonstrates the tremendous gains that can be realized for the patients when a systematic practice improvement approach to care redesign is embraced by the physician, health care staff, and organization.

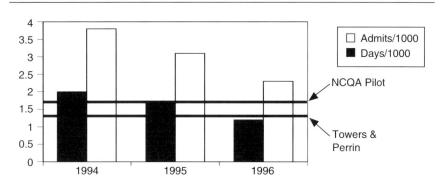

Figure 6–6 Plan Member (Ages 2–19) Asthma Hospitalizations per 1000 Plan Members (Ages 2–19). Courtesy of Lovelace Healthcare Innovations and Lovelace Health Systems, Albuquerque, New Mexico.

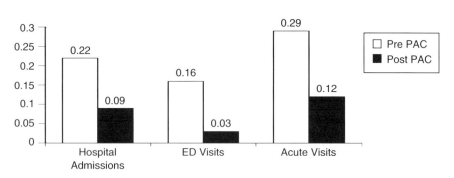

N = 86 patients followed for equal periods of time (9-month average).

Figure 6–7 Hospital, Emergency Department, and Acute Care Utilization per Patient before and after Initial Evaluation in the Pediatric Asthma Clinic. Courtesy of Lovelace Healthcare Innovations and Lovelace Health Systems, Albuquerque, New Mexico.

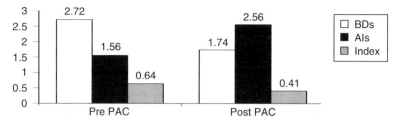

BD = Inhaled Bronchodilator; AI = Inhaled Anti-Inflammatory; Index = BD/(BD + AI).
N = 86 patients followed for equal periods of time (9-month average).

Figure 6–8 Inhaled Monthly Equivalents per Patient before and after Initial Evaluation in the Pediatric Asthma Clinic. Courtesy of Lovelace Healthcare Innovations and Lovelace Health Systems, Albuquerque, New Mexico.

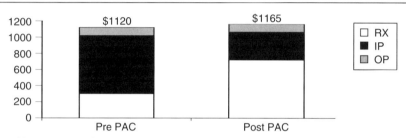

N = 86 patients followed for equal periods of time (9-month average).

Figure 6–9 Total Charges per Patient before and after Initial Evaluation in the Pediatric Asthma Clinic. Courtesy of Lovelace Healthcare Innovations and Lovelace Health Systems, Albuquerque, New Mexico.

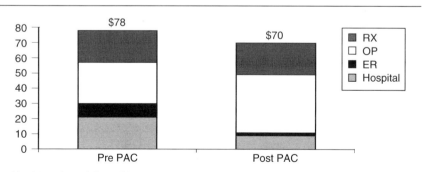

N = 86 patients followed for equal periods of time (9-month average).

Figure 6–10 Total Copayments per Patient before and after Initial Evaluation in the Pediatric Asthma Clinic. Courtesy of Lovelace Healthcare Innovations and Lovelace Health Systems, Albuquerque, New Mexico.

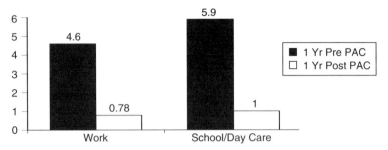

N = 45 patients reevaluated 1 year after PAC initial evaluation.

Figure 6–11 Days per Patient Lost Due to Asthma during Year before versus Year after Initial Evaluation in the Pediatric Asthma Clinic. Courtesy of Lovelace Healthcare Innovations and Lovelace Health Systems, Albuquerque, New Mexico.

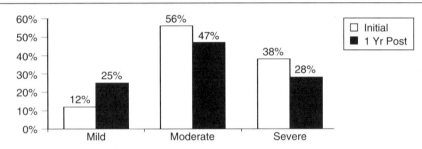

N = 45 patients reevaluated 1 year after PAC initial evaluation.

Figure 6–12 Asthma Severity at Initial Evaluation in the Pediatric Asthma Clinic and at Follow-up 1 Year Later. Courtesy of Lovelace Healthcare Innovations and Lovelace Health Systems, Albuquerque, New Mexico.

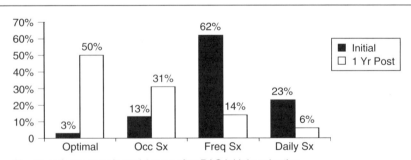

N = 45 patients reevaluated 1 year after PAC initial evaluation.

Figure 6–13 Asthma Control at Initial Evaluation in the Pediatric Asthma Clinic and at Follow-up 1 Year Later. Courtesy of Lovelace Healthcare Innovations and Lovelace Health Systems, Albuquerque, New Mexico.

SUMMARY AND ADDITIONAL LESSONS LEARNED

As illustrated in the case examples above, multiple implementation strategies are used within each EOC™ program. The strategies also vary from one program to the next. There is no cookbook or standard approach that works for every disease state. However, we have identified several common themes to consider when developing and implementing interventions in addition to those above.

The best implementation strategies are those that are simple and straightforward. As we all know, the enemy of the good or the excellent is the perfect. Lovelace's mantra is: Keep it SIMPLE! Unfortunately this is hard to learn, but is a critical element of the EOC™ design. Lovelace too has erred by making things too complicated and fancy in an effort to impress. These efforts always fail.

Dr. Bill Abeyta, a well-respected physician leader at Lovelace, offers another frequently overlooked design rule: "Do not create more work for the providers of care." The central tenet of quality improvement is to improve the processes and efficiency of systems. If this is accomplished, work flow should improve while providers' jobs become easier and more efficient. If an intervention creates more work, it will not be implemented by front-line staff.

Practice guidelines should not be a central focus. Rather, we should remember one of the more important observations made by Dr. Eddy: "If you can't measure it, you can't manage it." In the cases discussed above, practice guidelines were never presented as a central focus of implementation. Rather, they were considered to be one building block in the foundation of an entire disease management program. They were always a part of the program, but rarely the most important or largest piece.

The Lovelace strategy focused on the critical patient data while reporting them back to the people who manage the patient care process. The diabetes EOC™ interventions and reports are excellent examples of this strategy. When useful information is put in the hands of physicians, the caregivers who direct the process of care, dramatic improvements in care delivery will occur.

References

1. Nash D. Editorial: making it happen. *J Outcomes Manage.* 1996;3(3).
2. Gunter M, Byrnes J, Shainline M, Lucas J. Improving outcomes through disease specific clinical practice improvement teams: the Lovelace EPISODES OF CARE™ disease management program. *J Outcomes Manage.* 1996;3(3):10–17.
3. Byrnes J. Lovelace's innovative disease management program. *J Am Med Group Assoc.* 1996; 45(4):24–27.
4. *Albuquerque Tribune.* November 4, 1994.

5. Byrnes J, Shainline M, Lucas J, Gunter M. Lovelace Health Systems: restructuring for quality. In: Boland P, ed. *Redesigning Healthcare Delivery*. Berkeley, Calif: Boland Healthcare; 1996:482–501.

6. Lucas J, Gunter MJ, Byrnes J, Coyle M, Friedman N. Integrating outcomes measurement into clinical practice improvement across the continuum of care: a disease-specific EPISODES OF CARE™ model. *Managed Care Q*. 1995;3(2):14–22.

CHAPTER 7

Disease State Management in Managed Care Organizations

Robert E. McCormack

Disease state management represents the beginning of a change in the paradigm for health care. In the old paradigm, health problems were thought of as relatively unpredictable occurrences of acute simple (single-cause) disease financed by a risk-based insurance mechanism. Care was reimbursed on a per-service basis provided by single, isolated providers and evaluated as point-in-time episodes.[1] In the new paradigm, managed care organizations (MCOs) are moving to address chronic complex illnesses across the continuum of care in a population-based approach.

The driving force behind this movement to disease management (DM) is the need for improved cost-effectiveness. MCOs have had a definite impact on the cost of providing medical care in the United States. Much of their success to date has relied on negotiating prepaid, capitated agreements with hospitals and health care providers. By changing incentives, the MCOs have had a major impact on the cost of services. Initially, this cost savings was enough to propel managed care to the forefront of needed health care reform. Unfortunately, these managed care changes in incentives have not stopped the acceleration of overall health care expenditures in the United States. After the initial drop in cost as MCOs enrolled membership, medical costs began to rise again and have continued to rise at rates that exceed the rate of inflation. Recent reports do indicate that nationwide, health insurance premiums of health maintenance organizations (HMOs) have increased at a rate lower than inflation (0.5% in 1996) for the first time in close to a decade.[2] This is certainly an encouraging sign, especially since 1996 marked the year when 33% of Americans were enrolled in HMO insurance programs, making HMOs the most common type of health insurance in the United States. Still, this statistic is probably at least partly a reflection of the extreme competitiveness and price sensitivity in the HMO industry, not a result of actual reduction in medical costs.

The ability to address the specific costs of purchaser groups can be an important factor in a disease state management program. Evaluations of potential cost savings for a specific population show substantial opportunity. By extrapolating cost savings from clinical studies, it is possible to estimate actual cost savings for a given population. MCOs have recognized the potential marketing advantages of this approach to large employer groups.

The potential cost savings in a disease state management program are substantial. Based on statistical analysis of demographic information, the projected cost savings for a moderate-size MCO implementing successful disease management programs with total paid claims of $9 million per year are up to $300,000.[3] The largest potential savings for a specific DM program will vary with the characteristics of the population. An MCO with a large pediatric population will probably benefit from an asthma DM program, whereas an organization with an older population will probably benefit most from DM programs for cancer or heart disease (Figures 7–1 through 7–6).

Another driving force behind DM programs is the need to demonstrate effective, population-based quality improvement to meet regulatory demands and to address public concerns. A study published in October 1996 showed that chronically ill Medicare patients treated in HMO settings were almost twice as likely to see their health decline as their fee-for-service counterparts.[4] This study hypothesizes that cost-cutting measures by MCOs may be compromising the health of chronically ill patients. Establishing effective DM programs for chronically ill patients, as discussed in Chapter 1, and measuring outcomes are effective responses to this public concern.

An operational DM program has clear potential to allow an MCO to meet many of the quality improvement standards of the National Committee for Quality Assurance (NCQA), the leading accreditation body for MCOs in the United States. NCQA standards call for chronic disease–specific outreach programs that include the entire population at risk. Other NCQA standards call for demonstration of the effectiveness of clinical quality and service improvement activities.

Several specific NCQA standards can be met using DM programs. The most obvious is the requirement to identify members with chronic conditions and offer appropriate services and programs to assist in managing their conditions. The MCO has to identify at least two chronic conditions, implement programs that address the continuum of care for these conditions, identify and contact the appropriate members with the conditions, and measure the effectiveness of the health management program.

The critical NCQA requirements for demonstrating appropriate monitoring of performance against clinical guidelines, developing interventions and follow-up for clinical improvement, and demonstrating the effectiveness of activities under-

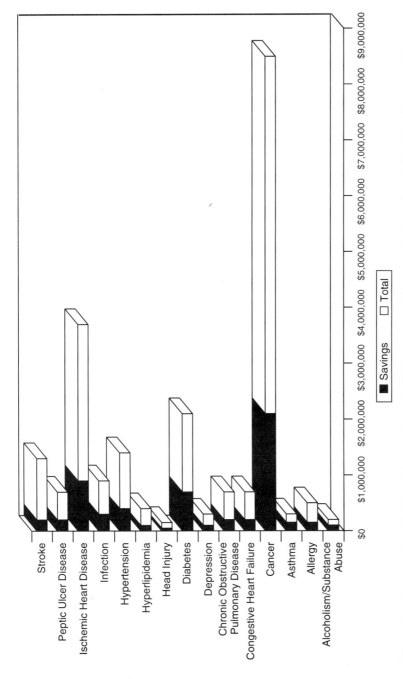

Figure 7–1 Retrospective Medical Claims Analysis of 1995 Data on Total Costs and Savings Potential for Most Frequent Diagnoses. Courtesy of Eris Survey Systems, Inc., Indianapolis, Indiana.

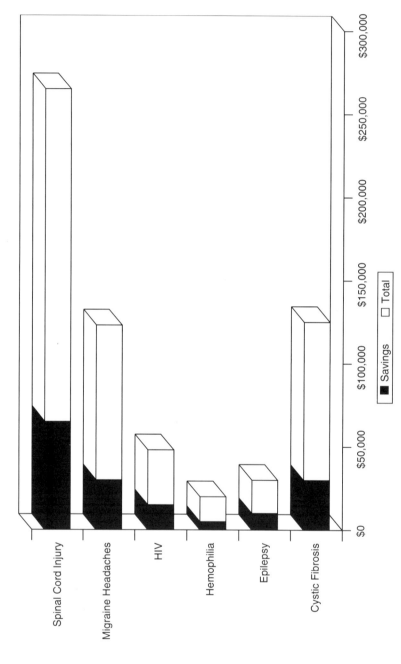

Figure 7–2 Retrospective Medical Claims Analysis of 1995 Data on Total Costs and Savings Potential for Infrequent but Costly Diagnoses. Courtesy of Eris Survey Systems, Inc., Indianapolis, Indiana.

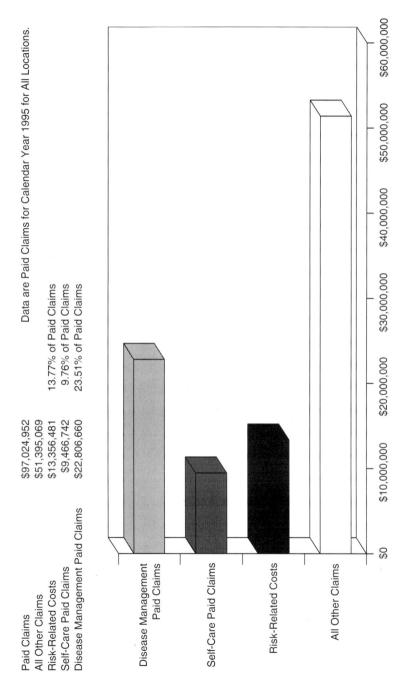

Figure 7–3 Retrospective Medical Claims Analysis of 1995 Data on Distribution of Claims Dollars. Courtesy of Eris Survey Systems, Inc., Indianapolis, Indiana.

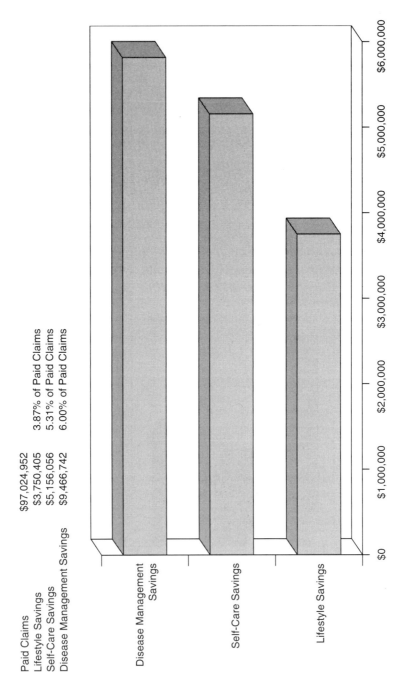

Figure 7–4 Retrospective Medical Claims Analysis of 1995 Data on Distribution of Potential Savings. Courtesy of Eris Survey Systems, Inc., Indianapolis, Indiana.

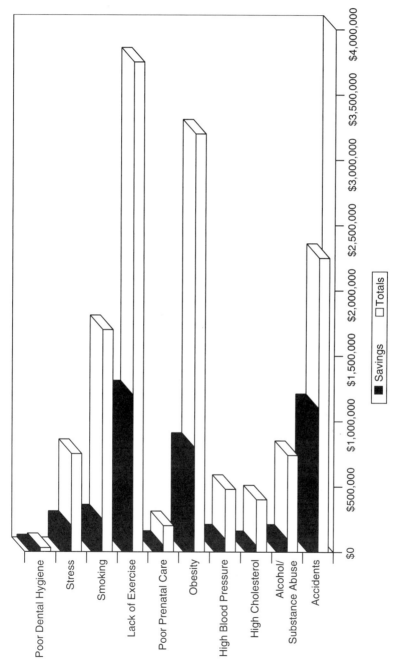

Figure 7–5 Retrospective Medical Claims Analysis of 1995 Data on Potential Savings from Disease Management Program Targeting Lifestyle and Behavior. Courtesy of Eris Survey Systems, Inc., Indianapolis, Indiana.

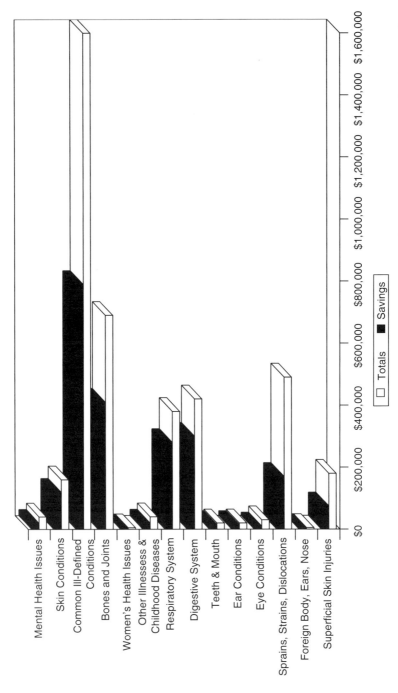

Figure 7–6 Retrospective Medical Claims Analysis of 1995 Data on Potential Savings from Disease Management of Various Conditions. Courtesy of Eris Survey Systems, Inc., Indianapolis, Indiana.

taken to improve clinical care can all be addressed through well-designed DM programs.

HEDIS

DM programs can also be used to improve performance measures on the Health Plan Employer Data and Information Set (HEDIS), a national measurement program started in 1993 and operated by NCQA. This program is attempting to develop a voluntary reporting system that allows employer groups and consumers of health care to compare MCO performance in key quality and utilization areas. The measurements evaluate population-based utilization rates of MCO members receiving pediatric immunizations, annual diabetic eye examinations, and beta blocker usage after myocardial infarction. The most recent version of HEDIS, called HEDIS 3.0, also includes a measurement of Medicare member functional status (the SF-36).

Most MCOs would not choose to develop a comprehensive DM program based on HEDIS alone, since HEDIS measures tend to be very focused. Still, a diabetes DM program could clearly be helpful in improving the rate of annual diabetic eye examinations. A DM program focused on heart disease could address the use of beta blockers after myocardial infarction. Clearly, an MCO will want to look at its HEDIS results when developing DM programs.

HISTORY OF DM IN MCOs

Until recently, with few exceptions, MCOs' fundamental approach to the management of costly medical conditions had changed very little over 10 years. To address the acceleration of medical costs and the increasing price competition in the market, many MCOs have now turned to DM.

MCOs have traditionally operated separate programs to address

- *Clinical quality improvement and utilization management:* guidelines for cost-effective, optimal disease treatment/management
- *Education:* improving members and provider knowledge about management of disease and member risk behaviors
- *Case management:* hospital-based, ambulatory care–based and home health care–based treatments/interventions

DM in MCOs combines these traditional programs of an effective MCO in a comprehensive long-term approach to improving member health and optimizing cost-effectiveness. This new approach fundamentally changes the way chronic disease conditions are managed.

CURRENT DM PROGRAMS IN MCOs

Because MCOs already have quality improvement, utilization management, member education, and case management programs, defining what represents a DM program in a managed care setting can be confusing. An MCO that develops a clinical guideline, educates members and providers about the guideline/disease, and measures outcomes is not necessarily operating a DM program. All of these traditional MCO areas are necessary components of a true DM process. But more than that, these areas must be coordinated over time to operate effectively across the entire continuum of the disease for the MCO's entire population at risk. The program must address more than just an isolated episode of disease; it must address the whole patient within the context of his or her disease process, including the home environment. MCO's are only beginning to use the full potential of their health care delivery systems through this comprehensive DM approach. The operational components of DM in MCO are shown in Exhibit 7–1.

Data Systems

A critical component for success in a DM program is complete and accurate data. The MCO must be able to identify the population at risk, track it over time, and measure the effectiveness of interventions. It cannot address the needs of a population unless it can find them. The modern term for this type of data system is informatics.[5]

MCOs should excel at these types of data-driven programs. Unfortunately, most of the data systems in MCOs were originally designed to track claims rather than to integrate clinical and cost data from multiple sources into a readily accessible format. As a result, much of the data needed to operate successfully a DM

Exhibit 7–1 Operational Components of MCOs' DM Programs

- Accurate data systems (population identification, tracking, financial and utilization information)
- Identification of a chronic disease management opportunity
- Guidelines outlining optimum DM
- A system to educate providers about the DM program and to obtain buy-in
- A system to assess members at risk to allow early interventions
- Clinical interventions based on guidelines
- Appropriate interventions across all care settings (home, office, hospital)
- Outcomes information on both cost and quality linked to the DM program activities

program must be identified on multiple databases or from paper sources and manually pulled together.[6] Most of the MCOs in the United States are attempting to create data "warehouses" from their existing databases in an attempt to link them together and allow easier access to data. This is clearly an interim step on the road to an integrated (computerized) medical record. Unfortunately, the barriers to the widespread use of integrated medical records are substantial and will probably not be overcome anytime soon.

However an MCO obtains the data, it is important to look at the membership population to confirm that there are enough members with a chronic disease condition to warrant the time and expense of designing and implementing a DM program. This type of analysis is also important to establish if the population is large enough to allow statistical validation of results. If, for example, an MCO has only 150 diabetic members, it may be statistically impossible to demonstrate a valid improvement in outcomes because the population is too small to have enough statistical "power." Data systems also allow analysis of data related to outcomes, both clinical and financial. Pending the development of an affordable and reliable integrated medical record system, MCOs are generally forced to supplement automated data with data that are manually abstracted from paper medical records. Data extraction from medical records raises questions about inter-rater reliability and is very costly. Data pulled from claims databases are prone to multiple errors. Trying to obtain any accurate information about outcomes is difficult, if not impossible, due to the simplistic nature of most of the data extracted by these methods. The data usually are not adjusted for case mix or severity of illness either. Conclusions about the significance of outcomes based on these types of data systems need to be made with caution.

Identification of Chronic Disease Management Opportunities

The identification of a chronic disease state with opportunities for improvement is very important. Most of the DM programs operating in MCOs address chronic illnesses that are relatively common in the general population and/or have a high cost of treatment. These existing programs include such conditions as asthma, diabetes mellitus, congestive heart failure, chronic renal failure, high-risk pregnancy, hypertension, and heart disease. These are all medical conditions with evidence that improved medical management will affect outcomes (see Table 7–1). In general, improved outcomes should result in reduced cost of treatment and improved quality of life. The reduced cost of treatment is an important aspect of these programs, since they can be relatively expensive to design and operate. It is important that these medical conditions have evidence of wide variation in treatment, which represents an opportunity for improvement. Payer concerns are also important. Medical conditions that affect payer cost and decrease absenteeism as

Table 7–1 Medical Conditions with Known Potential for Improvement

Disease State Management Condition	Opportunity
Congestive heart failure	Use of angiotensin-converting enzyme (ACE) inhibitors, early identification of decompensation with aggressive home treatment
Pediatric asthma	Use of inhaled corticosteroids, improved self-management, early identification of decompensation with aggressive home treatment
Diabetes mellitus	Tight glucose control, intensive member education, aggressive monitoring for early complications
Cardiovascular disease (high blood pressure, atherosclerotic heart disease)	Lifestyle interventions (weight, lipids, exercise, smoking cessation), medication compliance
Renal failure	Early identification for shunt placement, intensive member education and follow-up
Maternal/child health	Early identification of high risk pregnancy, aggressive treatment protocols, neonatal home care

well as improve quality of care will be well received by payers. This is a significant marketing consideration.

A good example of this type of strategy is Lovelace Health Systems' selection of 14 medical conditions for DM (see Chapter 6), nine of which (shown by asterisk) represented 24% of all the cost of care at Lovelace[7]:

1. diabetes*
2. pediatric asthma*
3. coronary artery disease*
4. pregnancy/birth*
5. low back pain*
6. breast cancer*
7. stroke*
8. knee care*
9. depression*
10. congestive heart failure
11. adult asthma
12. Alzheimer's disease

13. hysterectomy
14. attention deficit disorder

Guidelines for Optimal DM

The guidelines needed to implement DM in an MCO do not have to be complicated. They do need to include critical educational and lifestyle components for the members and critical clinical components for providers. Many of the organizations implementing congestive heart failure DM programs rely on an abbreviated version of the clinical practice guideline for heart failure published by the Agency for Health Care Policy and Research (AHCPR).[8] An article published in April 1996 details the consensus process used by RAND to develop review criteria based on the heart failure guideline.[9] This process resulted in the reduction of 34 recommendations to eight criteria with suggested compliance goals.

Diabetes mellitus DM programs most frequently rely on the published recommendations of the American Diabetes Association[10] and the findings of the Diabetes Control and Complications Trial Research Group (DCCT).[11] Asthma programs most frequently use National Institutes of Health recommendations.[12]

To succeed, the DM programs must have clearly defined goals that are accepted by members, providers, and the DM support personnel. The only way to optimize treatment is to articulate expectations clearly. For example, the goals of the Staged Diabetes Management Program developed by the International Diabetes Center in Minneapolis include diabetes treatment goals based on the patient's blood glucose and HbA1c levels.[13] The worse the diabetic control is, the more intensively the patient is managed by a combination of physicians, nurses, and registered dietitians. The program includes an algorithm for optimal management. The preliminary results of this program are encouraging, with mean HbA1c reductions from 0.6% to 2.4% over a 1-year period.

A System To Educate Providers about the DM Program and To Obtain Buy-in

Buy-in from plan providers is critical to the success of a DM program in an MCO. The program should be seen as supporting and augmenting provider management of the patient with a chronic disease, not supplanting it. Providers should be sent information on their patients and should receive regular communications from case management nurses on their patients' progress. A provider orientation to the DM program should be done as early in the process of implementation as possible. Physicians will be resistant to any program that they perceive will increase their paperwork or daily responsibilities. Physicians and other practitioners need to have input into the DM process to ensure that the program will meet their needs and not adversely affect their office practice. In an independent practice association (IPA) network setting primary care physicians may need reassurance that the patients enrolled in the program will still feel that they are being managed by their physician and not by the MCO's DM program.

It is important that physicians see a gap between what they think they are doing in a clinical area and what they are actually doing that matters to a patient. Benchmarking plan data against other physicians' best-practice performance data is an effective tool to create a tension for change. Much of physicians' behavior is based on habit and their perception of the effectiveness of a given therapy or process. To change their behavior, physicians need concrete, scientific evidence that a different therapy or process is more effective than their current practice. This type of benchmarking against best practices also demonstrates that better performance is possible. Someone else has done it better. When followed up by education on what the physician needs to do to close that gap, this can be a highly effective tool. Follow-up with outcome information showing that patient care has improved reinforces the change.

It is also very helpful to pilot an untested program on a limited basis to obtain internal benchmarking information, as well as to identify any problems with the process before it is fully implemented. Attempting to roll out a DM program before a pilot has been done can result in problems that destroy the credibility of the program with providers, members, or both. A successful pilot can be very useful in obtaining buy-in from an MCO's physicians and other practitioners.

A System To Assess Members at Risk To Allow Early Interventions

MCOs are identifying high-risk members in several ways. The most common is using claims data based on hospital admissions, length of stay, emergency department (ED) visits, and overall paid claims for a given group of members with an identified disease condition. For example, members with congestive heart failure who have been admitted in the prior year are probably at higher risk than patients with this condition who have never been hospitalized. In fact, the stage of congestive heart failure seems to correlate directly with the risk of hospitalization.

Another method of quantifying patient risk is the use of a survey or questionnaire. This is particularly helpful when lifestyle issues are important. In some MCO programs, these surveys are used to identify risk factors as well as to attempt to measure reduction in risk for members enrolled in a program. In the Humana Cardiovascular Health Improvement Process (CHIP) for hypertension, all members identified with hypertension were sent a cardiac risk check questionnaire to help the members, their providers, and the health plan identify members who were at increased cardiac risk.[14] Once these risks were identified, the program works with the members to reduce or change those risks that are modifiable. Repeating the risk assessment over time can help quantitate the effectiveness of the program's interventions (see page 187).

In some instances, the diagnosis of the disease itself is an issue. For example, this type of risk assessment tool can be applied to attention deficit hyperactivity disorder (ADHD). This condition is difficult to diagnose, and the diagnosis can be expensive to establish. A simplified tool has been developed that both reduces the cost and improves the accuracy of the diagnosis of ADHD.[15] This tool is designed to be administered by the primary care physician and cuts the cost of screening for ADHD from approximately $0.64 per pediatric member per month to $0.19 per pediatric member per month.

Clinical Interventions Based on Guidelines

To be successful, a DM program must have a clinical road map to follow. The clinical recommendations can be relatively simple, but they need to cover all critical aspects of the disease process, including lifestyle issues as well as clinical management issues. A quality improvement guideline is the most common method of approaching this need. The guideline may be as simple as a series of recommendations that will be implemented through the DM program. For example, a program for congestive heart failure (CHF) would probably include a recommendation that members without contraindications be on angiotensin-converting enzyme (ACE) inhibitors. ACE inhibitors have been demonstrated to reduce both morbidity and mortality for patients with congestive heart failure. Additional critical components would need to be identified and implemented. In the RAND Consensus Group, eight other criteria were identified from the original 34 recommendations of the AHCPR guideline (Exhibit 7–2). From the guideline, critical areas for monitoring and building a member and provider education program, measurements, and interventions to improve both quality of care and cost may be identified.

Appropriate Interventions Across All Care Settings

This is a critical component of a successful DM program. Interventions not only should include all of these settings but should include them repetitively, as needed over time, rather than in response to an isolated episode of illness. The primary goal of these interventions is to prevent or reduce the severity of an episode of illness.

These interventions can take many forms. Most DM programs in MCOs seem to be following one of two basic forms. The first form may be called the *case management model*. These programs have a nurse or other appropriate health care professional dedicated to the long-term follow-up of chronically ill patients. This

Exhibit 7–2 Quality Criteria Adapted from AHCPR Guideline for Congestive Heart Failure

---

1. All patients with a diagnosis of heart failure should have received an initial assessment of left-ventricular function by echocardiography, radionuclide ventriculography, or contrast ventriculography. The result should be documented in the record.
   Standard of Quality: 90%–95%

2. At each visit for heart failure, patients should have the following items documented:
   a. Blood pressure
   b. Weight
   c. Symptom status, including whether they are better, worse, or the same as at the previous visit
   d. Assessment of volume overload, including mention of the presence or absence of at least one of the following: third heart sound, rales, jugular venous distention, peripheral edema
   Standard of Quality: 90%–95%

3. If clinical evaluation and/or chest radiography showed evidence of volume overload (that is, leg edema, ascites, rales, jugular venous distention, or pulmonary edema), the patient should be receiving a diuretic.

4. All patients with LVEF <=35% should be receiving an ACE inhibitor unless there is documented intolerance or contraindications to ACE inhibitors or the serum potassium has been greater than 5.5 at a time when the patient was not taking potassium supplements or a potassium-sparing agent. The dose of the ACE inhibitor should be at least
   a. 10 mg BID of enalapril
   b. 50 mg TID of captopril
   c. 20 mg QID of lisinopril
   d. 20 mg BID of quinapril
   Reasons for smaller doses should be documented.
   Standard of Quality: 90%–95%

5. A record should appear that at the time of initial diagnosis or assessment the patient received counseling concerning the importance of diet, daily weights, and compliance with treatment recommendations.
   Standard of Quality: 90%–95%

6. If patients experience persistent or worsening symptoms and/or signs of volume overload, a record should appear that they were questioned concerning their com-

continues

Exhibit 7–2 continued

pliance with diet and medications. Such questioning need take place only periodically, for example, every 6 months.
Standard of Quality: 90%–95%

7. If patients experience persistent or worsening symptoms and/or signs of volume overload despite compliance with medications and diet, one of the following should be documented:
   a. A diuretic was newly prescribed.
   b. The dose of the diuretic was increased.
   c. A loop diuretic was initiated in a patient previously taking a thiazide diuretic.
   d. A second diuretic (such as spironolactone) was added to the regimen of a patient taking a loop diuretic.
   e. The patient was admitted to the hospital for intravenous diuretic therapy.
   f. It is stated that the patient cannot tolerate a higher dose of diuretic because of hypotension or renal insufficiency.
   Standard of Quality: 75%–80%

8. Patients should not have received more than one measurement of left-ventricular function unless one of the following is documented as the reason for the second (or subsequent) test:
   a. New heart murmur
   b. New myocardial infarction
   c. Sudden deterioration despite compliance with diet and medications
   d. Progressive symptoms possibly requiring heart transplant
   Standard of Quality: 75%–80%

Source: © *Journal on Quality Improvement.* Joint Commission on Accreditation of Healthcare Organizations, 1996, pp. 265–276. Reprinted with permission.

nurse either sees the patients at their homes or telephones on a regular basis. In this type of DM program, based on the case management model, the patient helps develop his or her own long-term care plan, including an action plan for worsening disease symptoms (if appropriate). Home visits are typically an important part of this type of program and may include clinical examination and home treatment.

The second form may be called the *coordinated outreach model.* These programs rely primarily on pulling existing resources together, such as educational classes, written educational materials, and contracted health care providers, to create a better coordinated program for management of a chronic disease state. To qualify as a "true" DM program, there must be an identification of all members with the condition, a method of tracking their progress over time, a practice guideline, and a telephone and/or mail outreach program focused on the clinical goals for improving the utilization and quality of services provided.

Both of these forms have inherent advantages and disadvantages. In general, the case management model is most appropriate for a DM program that addresses a chronic disease with acute exacerbations, such as CHF. There, a home intervention can interrupt an acute exacerbation and potentially prevent hospitalization. The coordinated outreach approach tends to be more appropriate for chronic diseases such as high blood pressure, where an adverse outcome is not as likely to be prevented by a specific home intervention.

An effective DM program requires potentially costly interventions. These interventions may involve members, providers, or both. Most programs involve both member and provider interventions.

Member Interventions

Member interventions can take several forms. Among the most common are mailed educational materials focused on the disease being managed. These mailed materials may include reminders for such services as annual dilated eye exams or influenza vaccinations for diabetic members. To be most cost-effective, the mailings often contain both educational and reminder information. How effective mailed interventions are in the management of members with chronic diseases is still being debated among MCOs. To some extent, the effectiveness may depend on the socioeconomic status of the members. For example, mailed reminder and educational interventions sent to Medicaid members may be less effective, especially if the materials are not developed at an appropriate education level for this population. It is likely that many members, regardless of socioeconomic status, do not take the time to read educational materials. Some MCOs are using mailings associated with an important date, such as a birthday or a national health month, to increase the likelihood that members will read a mailing and take some action based on the contents. It seems likely that mail interventions will be more successful if the membership affected is motivated and accepts and understands the importance of the intervention.

The major advantage of mail interventions is that, in general, they tend to be relatively inexpensive compared to other alternatives. To include brochures or bulky materials, envelopes are required, as opposed to fold-over-and-fasten post cards. Probably the average cost of a mailing that includes relatively inexpensive materials still amounts to less than $1 per member.

Member education through a group or individual teaching program is another form of intervention in chronic DM programs. This can take the form of a one-on-one appointment with a health professional such as a nutritionist or nurse educator. These interventions tend to be the most effective form of education. They do require the availability of the services and the cooperation and time of the member. For younger populations that are still in the active work force, the time needed to attend these educational programs can be a barrier. Sometimes holding these programs in more convenient locations and times can overcome this barrier. It is important to talk to the members before making plans for these programs. An evening program tends to interfere with family time, and day programs tend to interfere with work. Members who have more generous work-leave policies are more likely to attend day programs. A program that is recommended by the member's provider is also more likely to have good attendance.

To attempt to overcome the barrier of time and location, some MCOs are beginning to experiment with home-based educational programs. These programs may be computer-based, interactive, or more passive educational mediums such as videotapes. They have the distinct advantage of allowing the member to choose when to view the materials. Their chief disadvantage is they may not allow the member to ask questions. They also may require equipment, such as a VCR or home PC to which all members may not have access.

Another variation on the home-based educational program that is becoming more common is having a health professional perform a home visit. The health professional is most commonly a nurse who can visit with the member and his or her family, provide individual education tailored to the member's needs and the level of understanding of his or her disease, and answer questions. In some programs the nurse may even go so far as to help the member go through his or her kitchen looking for food items that may not be appropriate. In the more aggressive programs, this home visit will also include an evaluation of the member's medications and his or her current level of function and symptoms. If the member is experiencing significant difficulties, the nurse can call the primary care physician from the member's home and obtain orders for changes in the member's medications or other treatments. This last intervention is most likely to be helpful in disease conditions subject to acute exacerbations, such as congestive heart failure or asthma. Physician support is critical for this type of intervention. Some physicians are highly resistant to patient treatment suggestions or requests from home nurses.

Telephone intervention programs have shown great potential. A recent randomized controlled study describes an automated telephone system that was effective in improving a population's hypertensive medication compliance and mean blood pressure levels compared to those of the control group.[16] Similar telephone intervention programs are currently being investigated for diabetes mellitus. The clear advantage to automated telephone interventions is their relatively low cost and patients' ability to access the system at times convenient to them. Directed telephone outreach programs, where a professional calls the patient, are more problematic. They tend to be costly and are not well accepted by some patients. Directed telephone interventions are particularly useful when an intervention is needed for patients who are geographically dispersed and the intervention is relatively straightforward.

Incentives are sometimes used to support a member intervention. The incentive is not, in and of itself, an intervention, but it may increase the chances that members will respond. For example, an MCO could mail materials to members reminding them of an important health test, such as an annual dilated eye examination. Early detection of diabetic retinopathy reduces the incidence of blindness in this population. The MCO could include a coupon good for the cost of the eye examination or for the waiver of a copay for some other service offered by the MCO after the eye examination is completed. Another similar intervention is the use of a punchcard that is punched once for every visit/test and, when completely filled, is exchangeable for goods or services. Drawings for prizes based on participation or completion of desired behavior are another possible incentive to support an intervention. Incentives will not succeed if the member does not understand and accept the importance of the intervention.

Physician Interventions

Physician interventions are most frequently educational. Continuing medical education (CME) programs can be developed to support the goals of the DM program. Many organizations arrange for a speaker to come and discuss important issues in the management of a disease condition. This can be effective but may be poorly attended by providers. This approach can also be relatively expensive and difficult to schedule at convenient times. At Humana Health Care Plans of Kansas City, the educational programs developed to support the implementation of DM programs have taken the form of videotape CME. This has the advantage of allowing the educational program to be repeated many times and at many locations convenient to providers. The cost of developing and producing the videotape is not significantly higher than the cost of arranging a large auditorium space and paying a speaker to address a provider audience. To obtain category one American Medical Association (AMA) CME credit, the plan contracted with a local teaching hospital to support the educational program.

Another important form of education for providers involves obtaining information about current levels of compliance with plan DM guidelines and comparing this performance to national benchmarks and/or desired levels of performance. A good example would be ACE inhibitor usage in congestive heart failure patients without contraindications to these medications. ACE inhibitors are independently associated with reduced numbers of complications and longevity in patients with congestive heart failure. By measuring the current usage of these medications for the members and feeding this information back to the providers, a plan may be able to increase provider awareness of the importance of these medications. This is most effective when the individual physicians can see their patients' results compared to their peers and/or other organizations.

Barriers to the Development of DM Programs

There are barriers to the development of effective DM programs in MCOs. Those already discussed include the limitations of data systems, the need for physician buy-in and support, and the need for measurable outcomes. Additional barriers include the cost of developing and implementing programs, the difficulty in measuring any savings, and overlap in DM programs.

Overlapping DM programs can create problems with coordination of care. This can occur when the MCO is operating DM programs in diabetes and congestive heart failure. If a member has both medical conditions, which program will be primarily accountable for the member? This creates problems when trying to measure cost savings and establish outcomes. It can also create problems with the data systems' integrity.

DM programs can be costly to develop. MCOs have several methods available to pay for these programs. They may choose simply to budget for the costs and absorb them as a part of the premium. The traditional capitation system is sometimes used. Basically, the MCO pays a vendor, such as a home health agency, a per-case rate. An alternative system involves risk sharing. In this situation, a vendor, usually an established DM company with an existing specialty health care network, agrees to manage a group of patients with a chronic illness. As part of the agreement, the total cost of caring for these members is estimated, and a certain reduction in the cost is required before the vendor receives any payment. If the vendor fails to reduce medical costs, then it loses money or has a reduced profit.

Pharmaceutical companies are actively working to develop and market DM programs for MCOs. This is, in part, a marketing strategy designed around the pharmaceutical companies' therapeutic products used to treat various chronic medical conditions. These programs are almost always based on the coordinated outreach model of DM programs discussed earlier. Some of these programs do not have sufficient interventions built in to qualify as true DM programs. On the other hand, some of these programs are well constructed and have considerable promise. The most promising of these programs were built, not with a focus on marketing a specific product, but rather primarily as a value-added service for MCOs.

Internal development of DM programs is time consuming and costly. Large MCOs with significant resources can certainly develop these programs. In general, an internally developed program cost will depend, in part, on how many members will be included and the decision on which model of DM to use, case management or coordinated outreach.

The CHIP at Humana in Kansas City

An example of an internally developed DM program is the Cardiovascular Health Improvement Process (CHIP) in Kansas City, Missouri. This DM program is a joint venture between Hoerst Marion Roussel (HMR) pharmaceutical company and Humana Health Care Plans. Program development began in early 1995 when a multidisciplinary team consisting of HMR and Humana employees began meeting. Humana was interested in improving members' cardiovascular health, and HMR was looking for a way to enhance its effectiveness in the health care marketplace. The team chose to focus initially on hypertension due to its prevalence in the Humana membership population and the perceived opportunity to affect the outcomes for this group of members.

The primary goal of the CHIP program, as developed by the team, was to get hypertensive patients more actively involved in the treatment and management of their medical condition through lifestyle changes and a periodic assessment of their health condition and risk. Through these lifestyle improvements and by working with Humana providers, the team hoped to improve the health and clinical quality of care of these members. Humana established a guideline for the management of hypertension in late 1995. Education of plan providers about the importance of this guideline was integrated into the work of the team.

The CHIP team used Humana claims and encounter data to identity Humana members with a diagnosis of hypertension. They eventually found that approximately 10% of the total population of the plan had this diagnosis. Further analysis showed that 25% of adults and approximately 50% of senior members had a diagnosis of hypertension. These numbers reflect the incidence of hypertension in the general population, a fact the team found very reassuring in respect to data system integrity.

The team evaluated a great deal of information about lifestyle changes and the impact of lifestyles on hypertension as well as cardiovascular disease in general. Additional effort went into research about methods of affecting and maintaining such changes. One of the more interesting concepts identified by the team was Prochaska's concept of the "change cycle," which emphasizes that a person has to be prepared to change before any change can occur and that most people go through this process several times before any change in behavior becomes permanent.

Another key concept developed by the team was the need to have an effective tool to measure members' cardiovascular risk. This ultimately resulted in the plan's contracting with an external vendor to process a scannable form and produce a health risk appraisal (HRA) report. The HRA and educational materials about hypertension are mailed to the members along with an invitation to participate in the CHIP program.

This health risk report is used to inform the member of his or her risk factors for heart disease, as well as to track the impact of risk modification on the population. To support lifestyle changes, the process asks each member to identify one lifestyle area the member wants to change and to set a short-term, accomplishable goal toward that change. The member is asked to sign a "commitment" to work on improving this area. Research has shown that signing a written commitment does improve the chance that the member will succeed. The plan provided educational classes and written materials to support whatever area the member selected. The team also designed periodic written and telephone interventions for members participating in the program.

Plan physicians were involved in the development of the program through a pilot at one of the plan's medical centers. In addition, the plan identified a videotape CME program on hypertension to educate plan providers about the hypertension guideline. The plan established baseline clinical performance by auditing random medical records of members with hypertension against the hypertension guideline. Providers were also educated about the plan's clinical performance.

The outcomes selected by the CHIP team included plan performance on the clinical guideline, the impact of the program on member risk (measured by the health risk appraisal), and the impact of the program on member education about hypertension. The team also assessed the impact of the program on medication usage patterns of the membership. At this time, only preliminary results of these outcomes are available (see Exhibit 7–3).

Outcomes Information Linked to DM Program Activities

Measurements of effectiveness may be specific or general and may include both utilization- and quality-based outcomes. In the best programs, specific utilization and quality outcomes such as hospital admission rates, length of stay, ED visit rates, per-case cost rates, and member functional status are reported. In others, the outcomes are more implied and may be as simple as a reduction in overall hospital costs. These less specific outcomes may make it difficult to establish with any certainty that the DM program was responsible for the cost and/or quality improvements.

Quality outcomes most frequently measured include health and functional status (Short Form 36 [SF-36]), member satisfaction, complication rates, mortality rates, and some form of intermediate outcomes. Intermediate outcomes include improved medication use (e.g., use of ACE inhibitors in congestive heart failure patients), improved medication compliance, improved screening rates, and improved lifestyle factors. These improvements are intermediate outcomes because they do not, in and of themselves, represent a benefit to the patient. Their benefit has to be inferred on the basis of results of historical clinical studies and probabil-

Exhibit 7–3 CHIP Progress to Date

Progress to Date
- As of September this year, 9,109 CRCs mailed and 3,890 returned . . . a 43% response rate.
- Initial analysis of the CRCs reveals that the most common health risk of respondents is being overweight and/or physical inactivity.
- Data collection for first-year postimplementation outcomes is in process (at the time of this writing).

Lifestyle/Behavior Costs and Savings Projections
Company XYZ—1995 data
Chart 6—All Lives

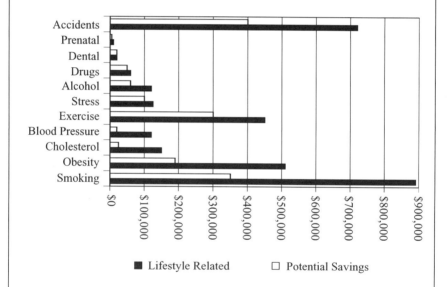

Courtesy of Hoechst Marion Roussel, Kansas City, Missouri, and Humana Health Care Plans, Kansas City, Missouri.

continues

Exhibit 7–3 continued

Disease Management Costs and Savings Projections

Paid Claims	$58,458,759	
DM Claims	$14,669,869	25.09% of Paid Claims
Male DM Claims	$8,380,903	57.13% of DM Claims
Male DM Savings	$2,093,184	24.98% of DM Claims

Selected Disease Management Savings for Males by Diagnosis

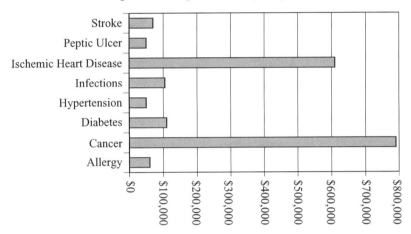

Cost
- Cost to develop program from scratch = $11.60 per member with HBP
- Cost per HBP member first year = $13.40
- Cost per HBP member each subsequent year = $12.00

continues

Exhibit 7–3 continued

Lifestyle/Behavior Costs and Savings Projections

Total Paid Claims	$58,458,760	
Total Lifestyle/Behavior		
Related Claims	$16,969,572	32.48% of Total Paid Claims
Male DM Claims	$8,734,131	45.99% of Total Lifestyle/
		Behavior Claims

Category	Totals
Accidents	$1,913,094
Alcohol/Substance abuse	548,629
High Cholesterol	206,997
High Blood Pressure	271,841
Obesity	1,373,476
Poor Prenatal Care	223,336
Lack of Exercise	2,597,255
Smoking	906,426
Stress	672,148
Poor Dental Hygiene	13,017
Total Savings	**$8,734,131**

continues

Exhibit 7–3 continued

Lifestyle/Behavior Costs and Savings Projections

Total Paid Claims	$58,458,760	
Total Lifestyle/Behavior Related Claims	$18,899,572	32.48% of Paid Claims
Lifestyle/Behavior Savings Potential	$8,734,131	45.99% of Total Lifestyle/ Behavior Claims
Lack of Exercise	$2,597,255	29.74% of Total Lifestyle/ Behavior Claims

Total Lifestyle/Behavior Savings Potential by Age Group

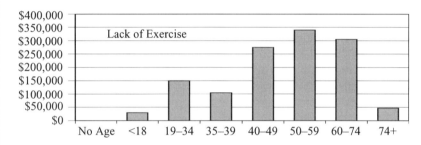

Lifestyle/Behavior Costs and Savings Projections

Total Paid Claims	$58,458,760	
Total Lifestyle/Behavior Related Claims	$18,899,572	25.09% of Paid Claims
Lifestyle/Behavior Savings Potential	$8,734,131	57.13% of DM Claims
Obesity	$1,373,476	24.98% of DM Claims

Selected Disease Management Savings for Males by Diagnosis

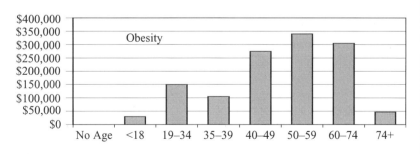

continues

Exhibit 7–3 continued

Lifestyle/Behavior Costs and Savings Projections

Total Paid Claims	$58,458,760	
Total Lifestyle/Behavior Related Claims	$18,899,572	32.48% of Paid Claims
Lifestyle/Behavior Savings Potential	$8,734,131	45.99% of Total Lifestyle/Behavior Claims
Smoking	$908,426	10.40% of Total Lifestyle/Behavior Savings Potential

Total Lifestyle/Behavior Savings Potential by Age Group

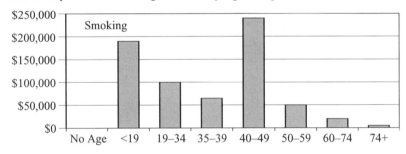

Lifestyle/Behavior Costs and Savings Projections

Total Paid Claims	$58,458,760	
Total Lifestyle/Behavior Related Claims	$18,899,572	32.48% of Paid Claims
Lifestyle/Behavior Savings Potential	$8,734,131	45.99% of Total Lifestyle/Behavior Claims
Stress	$672,148	7.70% of Total Lifestyle/Behavior Savings Potential

continues

Exhibit 7–3 continued

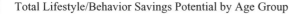

Total Lifestyle/Behavior Savings Potential by Age Group

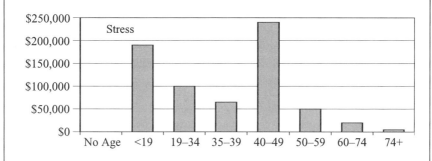

Lifestyle/Behavior Costs and Savings Projections

Total Paid Claims	$58,458,760	
Total Lifestyle/Behavior Related Claims	$18,899,572	32.48% of Paid Claims
Lifestyle/Behavior Savings Potential	$8,734,131	45.99% of Total Lifestyle/ Behavior Claims
High Blood Pressure	$271,841	3.11% of Total Lifestyle/ Behavior Savings Potential

Total Lifestyle/Behavior Savings Potential by Age Group

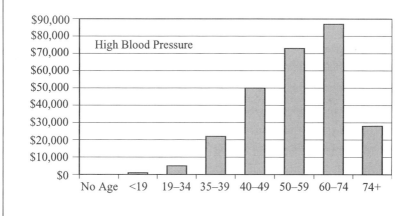

ity. For example, a patient who is obese and loses weight will probably live longer (but may not). A patient who has a screening test may be diagnosed earlier and statistically should have a better survival rate (but may not, especially if the screening test is incorrectly performed).

Intermediate outcome measures are used fairly frequently in DM programs due to the difficulty of establishing the relationship of true outcomes, such as mortality rates, with the activities of the DM program. For example, to establish with statistical certainty that an improvement in breast cancer screening rates at an MCO resulted in a lower mortality rate for female members would require a double-blinded sample of approximately 100,000 women followed for 10 years. It is much easier to establish that the screening rate has improved and to reference independent studies supporting the conclusion that fewer women in the plan will die of breast cancer due to the (implied) improved rates of detection. Another factor to consider is the confounding factors related to true outcomes measurements. While outcomes—mortality rates, for example—are being measured over time, the population being evaluated is getting older. Age is associated with higher mortality, so the mortality rates may go up because of this factor rather than because of an intervention being evaluated. A similar problem is encountered when assessing mortality rates based on where a patient has surgery. The mortality rates for any given hospital may vary on the basis of the severity of illness of patients at any given hospital. This confounding factor makes it difficult to judge hospital outcomes based solely on mortality rates without very sophisticated severity adjustment (see Chapter 4). Because of this, most organizations will continue to rely primarily on intermediate outcomes.

DM emphasizes continuous rather than episodic home care activities. In DM, individual members with chronic diseases are followed over time, with ongoing interventions even when they are doing well. This approach allows an MCO to work to reduce member risk, intervene before members become acutely ill, and reduce costly medical care in a systematic, thoughtful manner without adversely affecting outcomes. By measuring outcomes as part of a DM process, the MCO addresses the concerns of members, meets regulatory standards, and establishes that cost reduction does not equate with poor quality medical care. Effective DM programs hold the promise of finally addressing escalating health care costs for chronic medical conditions while actually improving the quality of care. MCOs are uniquely positioned to use their health care delivery networks to advance this process.

References

1. Pawlson G. Chronic illness: implications of a new paradigm for health care. *J Qual Improvement.* 1994;20:33–39.

2. KPMG Peat Marwick Employer Survey. 1996.

3. ERIS Survey Systems, Inc., Indianapolis, IN.

4. Ware JE, Bayliss MS, Rogers WH, et al. Differences in 4-year health outcomes for elderly and poor, chronically ill patients treated in HMO and fee-for-service systems. *JAMA.* 1996; 176: 1039–1053.

5. Sylvestri M. Health care informatics: the key to successful disease management. *Med Interface.* May 1996:94–99.

6. Brailer J, Kim L. From nicety to necessity: outcome measures come of age. *Health Systems Rev.* September/October 1996.

7. Lucas J, et al. Integrating outcomes measurement into clinical practice improvement across the continuum of care: a disease-specific episode of care model. *Managed Care Q.* 1995;3(2): 14–22.

8. Agency for Health Care Policy and Research. *Heart Failure: Evaluation and Care of Patients with Left Ventricular Systolic Dysfunction.* Available from AHCPR, PO Box 8547, Silver Spring, MD 20907. Clinical Practice Guideline No. 11, AHCPR Publication No. 94-0612.

9. Hadorn DC, Baker DW, Kamberg CJ, Brook RH. Phase II of the AHCPR-sponsored heart failure guidelines: translating practice recommendations into review criteria. *J Qual Improvement.* 1996;22:265–276.

10. American Diabetes Association. Standards of medical care for patients with diabetes mellitus. *Diabetes Care.* 1995;18(suppl 1):S8–S15.

11. Diabetes Control and Complications Trial Research Group. The effect of intensive treatment of diabetes mellitus on the development and progression of long-term complications in insulin-dependent diabetes mellitus. *N Engl J Med.* 1993;329:977–986.

12. National Heart, Lung, and Blood Institute. Guidelines for the diagnosis and management of asthma. National Asthma Education Program Expert Panel Report. *Pediatric Asthma, Allergy, Immunol.* 1991;5:57.

13. Ginsberg MD. Preliminary results of a disease management program for diabetes. *JCOM.* 1995;3(4):45–51.

14. ERIS Survey Systems 1996.

15. Heck E. Estimating prevalence and detection cost: prerequisites for disease state management of attention deficit hyperactivity disorder. *Am J Managed Care.* 1996;2:1175–1181.

16. Friedman RH, et al. A telecommunications system for monitoring and counseling patients with hypertension: impact on medication adherence and blood pressure control. *Am J Hypertension.* 1996;9(4):257–292.

CHAPTER 8

Disease Management in Pharmaceutical Companies

Harald Rinde

CHANGES IN THE HEALTH CARE MARKET

The concept of disease management was created in the early 1990s as a response to the need to contain health care costs while improving or maintaining the quality of patient care. The key factors fueling spiraling health care costs were

- an increasing elderly population
- increasing patient expectations and demand for quality and quantity of health care
- health insurance
- increased accessibility
- increase in new technologies
- increasing numbers of health care providers, including physicians
- lack of information on the cost-effectiveness of medical interventions in "real-life" settings
- lack of coordination and integration of health care components or elements, leading to duplications and inefficiencies

Throughout the world increasing health care costs were out of control. In the Unites States, health care spending reached 14% of the Gross Domestic Product (GDP). Though spending in other countries had not reached this high a proportion of GDP, health care costs were consuming huge resources in all countries. Figure 8–1 shows the growth of health care spending as a percentage of GDP in selected countries.

In the late 1970s, the focus shifted from improving health care (whatever the cost) to cost reduction. The initial attempts to contain costs were not very successful. One key reason for failure of many cost containment measures was the focus

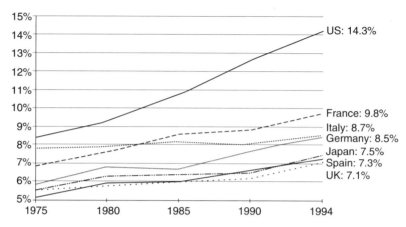

Figure 8–1 Total Health Spending As a Percentage of GDP. *Source:* Data from OECD, 1995.

on containing costs of isolated components of health care. The danger of this strategy is that restricting the use of one component often leads to increased use of other health care components. Cost savings may be demonstrated for that specific component, but in reality the cost has merely been shifted to other components. The result is that total health care costs may actually increase.

A study illustrating this cost shifting was conducted in the United States comparing health care costs in New Hampshire (N = 411) for low-income, elderly Medicaid patients using medications for chronic disease. A nearly identical patient population was used as control group in New Jersey (N = 1,375). New Hampshire introduced a cost containment measure, a cap on drug use. This cap restricted Medicaid schizophrenic patients to a maximum of three prescriptions per month. After 11 months, this measure was replaced with a $1 copayment per prescription. No cost containment measures were introduced in New Jersey. The cap in New Hampshire resulted in a 35% decline in drug use 11 months after the introduction of the cap. However, a simultaneous increase in admissions to nursing homes was observed. No changes were seen in the New Jersey control group. After the 11-month cap period, the drug use returned to nearly baseline levels, and the increased incidence of nursing home admissions ceased. In New Hampshire, 10.6% of the patients had been admitted to nursing homes after the 11-month cap period and 6.6% in New Jersey. The difference was highly significant, with a p value of 0.006. For the sicker patients, the percentages were 14.4% and 6.2%, respectively ($p = 0.0004$). The difference in admissions between the two groups is illustrated in Figure 8–2.

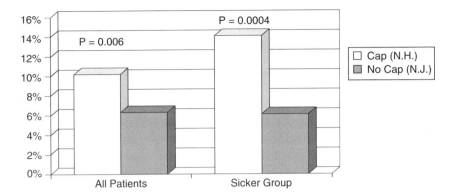

Figure 8–2 Nursing Home Admissions during the 11-Month Cap Period. *Source:* Data from S.B. Soumerai et al, *New England Journal of Medicine,* Vol. 325, No. 15, pp. 1072–1077, © 1991.

The savings from fewer drugs prescribed in New Hampshire during the 11-month period was estimated to be $300,000 to $400,000. This constituted a clear saving in one component of health care. However, the cost of the excess nursing home stay in the 11-month period was $310,745. Other additional cost items were not measured or included in the cost equation:

- excess nursing home stay after the 11-month period (90% of patients were still in a nursing home at the end of the 11-month period)
- excess care in nursing homes
- excess nursing home stay and hospitalization for populations not studied
- excess hospitalization (the difference between the two groups were not significant, but there was a moderate trend toward increased hospitalization in the New Hampshire [cap] group).[1]

This example illustrates how a measure restricting the use of isolated health care components results in a cost shifting and increase in total health care spending. It is essential to measure total spending across all health care components to measure adequately the effect of cost containment measures. However, with existing information systems, methods, and practices, it is rarely possible to do this properly. One of the core concepts of disease management is to permit the measurement of total cost for each disease across the relevant health care components, as illustrated in Table 8–1.

Table 8–1 Cost of Care

	Disease Management					Traditional
	G.P.	Hospital	Pharmaceut.	Other	Total	
Asthma	$xx	$xx	$x	$x	$xxx	
Diabetes	$xx	$xx	$x	$x	$xxx	
Hypertension	$xx	$xx	$x	$x	$xxx	
Epilepsy	$xx	$xx	$x	$x	$xxx	
Cancer	$xx	$xx	$x	$x	$xxx	
CHF	$xx	$xx	$x	$x	$xxx	
Total	$xxx	$xxx	$xxx	$xxx		

Another cost containment measure has been the introduction of managed care. The result has been a shift from fee for service, which stimulates more procedures, to capitation payment. The risk in a fee-for-service system is that patients are over-treated, whereas in a capitation system the risk is their being undertreated. Disease management attempts to strike a balance to ensure that patients receive optimal and cost-effective care.

CHANGING CUSTOMERS AND CHANGING NEEDS IN THE HEALTH CARE MARKET

Health care systems are rooted in a long history, and there is reluctance to change among the many players in health care, including physicians and health care policy makers. However, many shifts are occurring in the way health care is practiced and managed that will significantly change the health care environment. The changes in each country commence from different starting points, since each health care system is unique and different from the others. Some of the significant trends in health care throughout the world will both stimulate the need for disease management and be stimulated by disease management. These are

1. alignment of incentives
2. the need for physicians and other health care providers to deliver, measure, and demonstrate cost-effectiveness
3. the need for physicians and other health care providers to deliver, measure, and demonstrate quality services
4. the move toward evidence-based medicine (see Chapter 2)
5. demanding and increasingly informed patients

6. the emergence of on-line information and continuing education for physicians and other health care providers

Alignment of Incentives

In traditional fee-for-service health care systems, the various players have differing objectives. Patients want the best health care irrespective of cost. Physicians and other health care providers want to deliver as many services as they can charge. Payers want to pay for as little health care as possible. Health care policy makers want as much health care as possible within the limited budgets available. There is a need to align the objectives to ensure that optimal quality health care can be delivered from the limited resources available.

Various forms of managed care attempt to align the incentives. For example, in the United Kingdom, general practitioner (GP) fundholding groups (several GPs working together as a group in a geographical area) have control over almost the total health care budget. The payer, or purchaser, is also the provider; this ensures the alignment of incentives to provide efficient health care. Today, more than 45% of GPs in the United Kingdom belong to GP fundholding groups. In Switzerland, several health maintenance organizations (HMOs) have been established and are rapidly increasing their membership numbers. Isolated managed care organizations have been established in France, Italy, Spain, and the Netherlands. All European countries are currently discussing how to expand or establish various forms of managed care and how to align the incentives of key players in health care to ensure cost-effective health care delivery.

In many managed care organizations in the United States and Europe, physicians feel that their freedom to provide appropriate medical procedures and prescribe the appropriate medication is being restricted. Since there is an incentive to undertreat, patients may feel that they receive inadequate care. Managed care organizations have managed (somewhat) to align the incentives between payers and health care providers in terms of reducing cost. The challenge now is to balance this with improving quality of care and patient satisfaction.

The Need for Physicians and Other Health Care Providers To Deliver, Measure, and Demonstrate Cost-Effectiveness

As physicians' budget responsibility increases, the need to measure the cost-effectiveness of services becomes essential to identify which services add value. When physicians have budget responsibility, they need to measure how to get as much out of their limited budget as possible. In the United Kingdom, for example, fundholding GPs can invest surplus funds into their own practices. Payers must have a clear view of which services are the most cost-effective to manage their health care funds optimally. Managed care organizations need to minimize their costs while maintaining quality of care to stay competitive. In all cases, there is a need to capture and make intelligent conclusions from cost data. Costs must be measured across all health care components to optimize the overall care and avoid cost shifting.

The Need for Physicians and Other Health Care Providers To Deliver, Measure, and Demonstrate Quality Services

For most products and services, consumers, or institutional purchasers, usually have a range of sources of information that they can use to judge the quality of services or products. Reports that give the results from experts' analyses of products and services include restaurant and hotel guides, consumer reports on electronic equipment and reports on the best used cars to buy. However, when consumers or institutional purchasers buy health care services or products, there is little information available. Usually the buyer must rely on word of mouth based on individuals' personal experiences or on physicians' qualifications. This information is usually subjective and gives limited indication of the potential performance of the physician.

This is, however, beginning to change. In the United States, the National Committee for Quality Assurance (NCQA), an independent organization that provides "report cards," evaluates the quality of managed care plans. The Health Plan Employer Data and Information Set (HEDIS) currently contains 330 health plans in the United States (http://www.ncqa.org). The U.S. *Consumer Reports* publishes a quality ranking of HMOs, and *U.S. News and World Report* publishes a listing of the top 100 U.S. hospitals.[2] In the United Kingdom, the National Health Service (NHS) has published on the Internet the *NHS Performance Guide*. This guide lists all NHS Trusts and hospitals, GPs, and ambulance services, judged on a range of quality criteria (http://www.open.gov.uk/doh/tables96.htm). These readily available lists help consumers to make informed choices before seeking treatment. The great demand for such information on which to judge the quality of individual physicians or health care institutions will further stimulate its availability. To compete effectively in future health care markets, individual physicians, other health care providers, and institutions will need to supply objective information on quality. This will most likely be readily available to consumers and institutional purchasers.

To measure and demonstrate the quality of services, sophisticated information systems and processes need to be in place. Once the information has been captured, it needs to be analyzed for quality of care outcomes. The data will be used internally to improve the services on a continuous basis in addition to providing information to customers. Only exceptional health care providers have the capability of capturing and measuring outcomes today. There is a need for systems and services that can help this process along.

The Move Toward Evidence-Based Medicine

Physicians today largely base their decisions on personal experience and memory of best treatment from their original training or continuing education. There are different schools of thought concerning what appropriate treatments should be. Treatments vary from one physician to another and from one region to another. Faced with unusual or complicated cases, physicians are forced to make decisions based on limited information. They consult available written material or refer the patient to other physicians. The result is that the outcome of treatment of any one disease will be different depending on which physicians treat the patient or where the patient lives.

Recommended treatments today are almost exclusively based on well-controlled clinical trials. These trials are essential to determine if a new treatment is more effective or better tolerated than the established treatment. All variables not related to the questions to be answered need to be controlled. This is the method that has been used, and will be used in the future, to advance medicine. However, since these clinical trials do not adequately reflect real-life situations, in which variables cannot be controlled, the information gained from these controlled trials must be complemented by real-life outcomes measurements (see Chapter 4). The real-life data can be analyzed and used to develop best-practice guidelines (see Chapter 3). Through a continuous reevaluation of the process associated with certain outcomes, quality can continuously be improved. Physicians and other health care providers can thus practice evidence-based medicine based on real-life evidence. Evidence-based medicine has been defined as "the rigorous evaluation of the effectiveness of healthcare interventions, dissemination of the results of the evaluation and use of the findings to influence practice."[3] (See Chapter 2 of this book for a more extensive discussion.)

The collection, availability, and proper analysis of integrated real-life patient data for large numbers of patients are only in rare cases possible today. Some of the issues that limit the development of evidence-based medicine today are

- lack of information technology (IT) and its proper use when available
- differing IT platforms and standards
- lack of integration of IT
- lack of electronic patient data
- no universally accepted diagnostic and treatment coding

- the complexity of integrating all relevant data (clinical, pharmaceutical, cost, etc)
- patient confidentiality constraints
- the ownership of and accessibility to the appropriate data
- lack of expertise to analyze, make sense of, and make recommendations based on the measured outcomes

Evidence-based medicine is therefore today in its infancy. But it should become an essential tool for physicians to offer the best medicine for each specific patient and to provide the most cost-effective care for populations of patients.

Demanding and Increasingly Informed Patients

As baby boomers enter the age at which they become higher consumers of health care, they will be able to judge and will demand and expect high-quality services and products. The demand for and availability of health information have been steadily increasing over the years but have exploded with the development of the Internet and the World Wide Web. It has been estimated that there are more than 10,000 health-related sites on the Internet. In the United States, about 30% of cancer patients and about 50% of HIV-positive patients have used the Internet to access information.[4] An illustration of the power of the Internet as a channel for distribution of health information was the on-line conference for the launch of Rhone-Poulenc Rorer's (RPR) new drug Rilutek for the treatment of amyotropic lateral sclerosis (ALS or Lou Gehrig's disease). During a 2-hour period, RPR's Internet site was open for on-line chat with RPR's researchers, specialists, and patient advocates who were available to answer questions. During this 2-hour period, the site was visited by 14,000 interested parties.[5] The Internet is also a convenient medium for patients with similar interests and needs to conduct discussion groups and exchange information and experiences. Additionally, a wide range of CD-ROMs with comprehensive health information are available. Examples are *Medical Housecall*® and *Illiad*®, which provide detailed information about thousands of health-related conditions, medical hot lines and information services, cost analyses for treatments, and drug therapies in various geographical areas (see also Chapter 5).

This increased availability of health information is resulting in the consumerization of health care. It will empower patients to take a much more active role in managing their own health and in the clinical decision process. Patients will become more able to self-diagnose and self-treat and to challenge physicians' decisions.[2] To promote a healthy lifestyle, Pharmacia & Upjohn's disease management unit, Greenstone Healthcare Solutions, has launched an Internet-based free health risk assessment. The user answers about 40 questions and receives a personalized report with practical advice concerning how to improve health and pro-long life (http://www.youfirst.com/).

Through increasingly available information on the quality of physicians and other health care providers' services, patients are better able to select the best caregivers and treatments for them. John Wennberg found that when patients with prostate problems were given information about the disease and its treatment op-tions (on videodisks), they chose the least invasive, least costly options 70% to 80% of the time.[2] Surveys conducted in the United States by Louis Harris and the Institute for the Future found that about 20% of consumers were willing to pay themselves for health care that directly affected their well-being.[6]

There are several problems with health-related information:

- *The quality of the information.* Anyone can provide information on the Internet, and it is difficult to judge its quality and source. There is, therefore, a need for bodies that can filter and put some form of quality seal on the information.
- *The objectivity of the information.* Many providers of information have some interest in providing information that would lead to increased sales of prod-ucts or services. The pharmaceutical industry has much experience in provid-ing good health information. Pharmaceutical companies are, however, par-ticularly open to suspicion, since they have a self-interest. Frequently, the industry collaborates with independent organizations that can guarantee the objectivity of the information.
- *The availability and accessibility of appropriate information.* Searching the Internet usually results in hundreds or thousands of "hits," most of which are irrelevant. It is time consuming to find information on the Internet.

For these reasons, companies are emerging that can solve some of these prob-lems. For example, HealthGate Data (http://healthgate.com) provides a service allowing consumers and patients to search medical databases using lay-man's terms to get up-to-date information on research, clinical care, and drugs. HealthGate Data claims that they receive 30,000 inquiries per day and have over 4000 consumer accounts established.[2] Healtheon Corporation, formed by Netscape founder Jim Clarke, plans to provide an on-line health information service to patients to answer their questions.[2] These and other companies will emerge and will have a significant influence on consumers' demands, including the type of drugs they want.

Pharmaceutical companies are recognized as providers of high-quality educa-tional material. For example, Lilly Health Management Services (HMS), Lilly's disease management division, has launched diabetes education centers. These centers provide specialized education programs delivered by certified diabetes educators (registered nurses and dietitians) in convenient neighborhood locations.

The programs include information about the disease, lifestyle, diet, medication and so forth.[7]

Better-informed patients are more likely to become actively involved in the care process. This should improve compliance for prescribed treatment and necessary lifestyle changes. A better-informed general public will tend to follow healthier lifestyles and to adhere to the educational programs that are essential components of prevention programs. This in turn should improve the outcomes of health care in terms of quality and cost of care.

The Emergence of On-Line Information and Continuing Education for Physicians and Other Health Care Providers

Many types of information are necessary for making optimal clinical decisions. With existing and emerging technologies, critical information could become available to physicians at any point of care where physicians have access to a telephone line. Such electronic information might include

- *Patients' medical history.* Often the medical history is only partly known when important treatment decisions are made due to lack of available patient records. Through remote access, data stored in databases, on patients' "smart cards," or in electronic patient records could be accessed to enable physicians and other health care providers to make more informed decisions. Different health care providers would have access to the information they need to make the best decisions. The patient record could also be updated immediately with the new information.
- *Interactive decision-support systems.* On-line interactive systems could aid physicians in the diagnostic process. By feeding of information to a database, a list of most likely diagnoses and possible treatments could immediately be available at any point of care.
- *Best-practice clinical guidelines (based on outcomes analyses of large number of patients, using real-life data).* Once the diagnosis has been made, the best clinical treatment guidelines and the expected outcomes for that specific patient should be available on line.

An example of a system providing both electronic patient records and guidelines is Columbia/HCA Healthcare Corporation's planned network-based system that will enable physicians to access relevant information. The plan is to deploy personal digital assistants that will contain patient medical records, clinical guidelines, and outcomes information.[2]

Merck has created a searchable *Merck Manual* on its web site (http://www.merck.com/). The *Merck Manual* is probably the most used medical publication, both by health care professionals and by the general public. This service allows health care professionals to have instant access to information that will help them make better decisions about diagnosis and treatment and will eventually improve clinical outcomes for patients.

Physicians and other health care providers need to update their knowledge continuously to keep up to date with new therapies, drugs, and other developments. Today, this is mostly done through medical journals, conferences, books, and discussions with colleagues. This process is time consuming, and it is not possible to cover all necessary sources to gain the appropriate knowledge. New services are making information available to physicians on line. For example, Physicians Online Inc. (http://www.po.com) now claims 120,000 subscribers and 2 million e-mail messages exchanged per month. This service allows physicians to have access to and search for information at the desktop or at home in an efficient and time-saving manner. Many similar services will emerge, and technological development will allow more sophisticated services, including tailored information to be delivered directly to physicians' computers.

THE ROLE OF DISEASE MANAGEMENT

Disease management can be defined as a comprehensive, integrated, coordinated, and information-based approach to health care with the objective of continuously improving the value (quality-cost ratio) of patient care. Disease management will have a major influence on the way health care is practiced in almost all countries. The transformation caused by disease management will not be complete for many years. To facilitate disease management, information technology (IT) must be in place to capture and transmit data. It must be possible to make intelligent conclusions from the data. IT is at an early stage of development in the health care industry. It lags far behind that of other industries facing similar issues, such as the banking industry.

The introduction of disease management requires maintaining or improving the quality of care and customer/patient satisfaction while lowering or containing the cost of care. Instead of more products and services, customers expect delivery of value through health care services and products. The objective of disease management is therefore to identify and provide the health care that offers the *highest value and improvement in the quality-cost ratio*. In the search for the most efficient therapy, disease management is built on the idea of *continuous improvement*. Quality of care, quality of life, and satisfaction of customer needs will be measured, in addition to cost of care, before and after a health care intervention. The results of outcomes research will be analyzed and used to optimize interventions and to improve outcomes further. This continuous improvement process is illustrated in Figure 8–3. As new or modified interventions are introduced, real-life

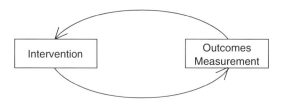

Figure 8–3 Disease Management: Continuous Improvement Process

outcomes will be measured to assess the value of the new intervention. Interventions can thereby be modified and improved continuously. This calls for the coordination and integration of all the various components of health care (prevention; primary, secondary, and tertiary care; home care; diagnostics; pharmaceuticals; etc) to achieve the most effective approach to health care and patient management. Interventions should improve the quality-cost ratio of patient care.

Further tools of disease management include

- *Clinical practice guidelines* (resulting from outcomes research and continuous improvement) to indicate to physicians and other health care providers optimal clinical practices
- *Utilization reviews,* eg, drug utilization reviews (to ensure appropriate use of interventions)
- *Support and education* of physicians, other health care providers, and patients to ensure optimal delivery of care and patient collaboration through knowledge of the disease and of patients' own responsibilities
- *Compliance management* to ensure that patients adhere both to therapy and to the lifestyle changes recommended by their caregiver

Particular targets for disease management are chronic diseases requiring long-term care of patients, such as asthma, diabetes, osteoporosis, epilepsy, cancer, and AIDS, and states such as menopause and aging.

DEVELOPMENT OF THE DISEASE MANAGEMENT CONCEPT

Disease management is most developed in the United States but is slowly establishing a foothold in other countries. Countries in which there has been some financial incentive alignment and budget responsibility, often with some form of managed care system, tend to be more open to disease management. Figure 8–4 illustrates the degree of openness to disease management in some key countries.

Disease management has evolved at various speeds in different countries and with different health care players. In all countries, pharmaceutical companies have been prime drivers along with local health care players:

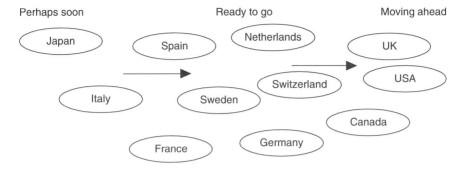

Figure 8–4 Openness to Disease Management. *Sources:* Data from H. Rinde; M. Hall, Promar International: Disease Management in Europe, 1995.

- In the United States, disease management has been driven primarily by managed care organizations.
- In the UK, it has to some extent been driven by the NHS, especially GP fundholding groups.
- In Germany, the "Krankenkassen" (the German health insurers) are the primary drivers of disease management.

In general, we can expect various forms of managed care and disease management to emerge, develop at different speeds, and coexist with other systems.

Disease management is an attractive proposition for all key players in health care. The "six Ps" of disease management are

1. *Patients,* who wish to receive better quality of care
2. *Physicians and other health care providers,* who wish to offer superior services for less cost and thus become more competitive
3. *Payers,* who wish to reduce health care costs
4. *Policy makers,* who wish to facilitate superior health care at less cost
5. *Pharmacists,* who wish to expand their role in the health care value chain
6. *Pharmaceutical companies,* who wish to form partnerships with customers and offer a wider spectrum of products and services

DOES DISEASE MANAGEMENT PRODUCE RESULTS?

Disease management is still in its relative infancy. Demonstrating the outcomes of disease management programs may take a long time. There are, however, some documented examples that demonstrate positive outcomes of programs.

The National Jewish Center in Denver, Colorado, is one of the leading medical centers for research and treatment of chronic respiratory diseases. Its "Time Out for Asthma" is a comprehensive disease management program for severe asthma patients. The program consists of a 5- to 7-day evaluation program involving a multidisciplinary team. The elements of the program are to

1. establish the diagnosis of asthma and exclude other forms of airflow limitations
2. identify factors that perpetuate the disease
3. determine optimal functioning levels for patients
4. agree on a medical regimen for optimal functioning with minimal side effects
5. educate patients on asthma, treatment programs, and self-management programs
6. address the psychosocial issues of a chronic disease with significant morbidity

The cost-related outcomes of the program 1 year after the program compared with base data are illustrated in Figure 8–5.[8]

There are many examples of the benefits of educational programs. Tables 8–2 and 8–3 provide a summary of several studies that measured the cost benefit and improvement in quality of care, including improvements in patient satisfaction from several educational programs.[9] Table 8–2 shows the results and cost savings from patient educational programs in managed care settings, and Table 8–3 shows these for programs in other settings.

From these studies Bartlett concluded that

- On average, for each $1 invested in patient education, $3 to $4 were saved.
- Less frequent complications and exacerbations were observed.
- Patients felt more confident in self-management of symptoms.

In other words, patient educational programs can be highly cost-effective and can improve the quality of care and patient satisfaction.

PHARMACEUTICAL COMPANIES AND DISEASE MANAGEMENT

As the practice of medicine is changing, so too must pharmaceutical companies. Companies may adopt a "wait-and-see" approach, since it will take time for the effect of some of the changes to become clear. Alternatively, companies can take a proactive approach and become actively involved in shaping the way health care will be practiced in the future. With so many changes in the market already taking

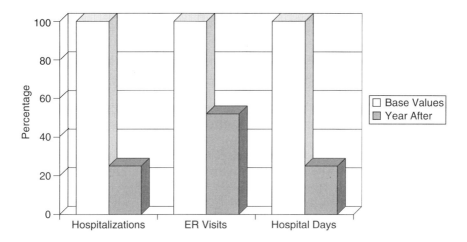

Figure 8–5 Outcomes Data from the National Jewish Center's Disease Management Program. *Source:* Data from W.E. Todd, *A Partnership Model for Asthma Disease Management,* National Jewish Center, presentation at Disease Management IIR Conference, January 25–27, 1995, Philadelphia, Pennsylvania.

Table 8–2 Benefits from Patient Education in Managed Care Settings

Author	Condition	Intervention	Results	Cost	Savings
Lewis et al	Asthma	Group education	Reduced ER use & hospitalization	$37/pt.	$217/pt.
Ershoff et al	Prenatal care	Nutrition counseling & smoking cessation	Reduced preterm births from 6.9% to 1.7%	$93/pt.	$183/pt.
Kemper	General	Self-care workshops	Reduced specialist referrals by 24%	$36/fam.	$55/fam.
Vickery et al	Minor illness	Self-help materials & counseling	Reduced visits for minor illnesses by 35%	$22	$77

Source: Data from E. Bartlett, *Cost-benefit analysis of patient education,* proceedings of the Patient Education Congress, June 1994.

Table 8–3 Benefits from Patient Education in Other Settings

Author	Condition	Setting	Results	Cost	Savings
Neresian et al	Diabetes	Public health dept.	Reduced hospitalization by 33%	$150/pt.	$442/pt.
Roberts et al	Upper respiratory infection (URI)	Clinic	Reduced URI visits by 29%	—	—
Lorig et al	Osteoarthritis	Community	Reduced pain by 20%, physician visits by 43%	$54/pt.	$189/pt.
Lorig et al	Rheumatoid arthritis	Community	Reduced pain by 20%, physician visits by 43%	$54/pt.	$648/pt.
Caudill et al	Chronic pain	Clinic	Reduced clinic visits by 36% in 1st year	$101/pt.	$312

Source: Data from E. Bartlett, *Cost-Benefit Analysis of Patient Education,* proceedings of the Patient Education Congress, June 1994.

place, all pharmaceutical companies are exploring what they should do to respond to these changes. One key strategy to address these changes and new demands in the market is to focus on disease management. All pharmaceutical companies have evaluated the possibility of embracing this strategy, and many are experimenting with, or have initiated, disease management activities.

Physicians and other disease management partners can benefit from several core competencies of pharmaceutical companies. Pharmaceutical companies have a range of core competencies that they are using in R&D and in marketing their products or in running and optimizing their core businesses. Many of these can be developed into services or products that can complement their core business or be the basis for new businesses. Some of these core competencies are discussed below.

Medical Knowledge and Understanding of Diseases

Pharmaceutical companies are in the forefront of medical R&D and have vast resources in house and an in-depth understanding of diseases and their treatments. Companies often have key people and large databases that could be leveraged in developing disease management programs.

Medical Opinion Leader Networks

In addition to in-house expertise, pharmaceutical companies have large networks consisting of key thought leaders around the world. These resources can be used in the development of several aspects of disease management programs. One example would be the development of clinical guidelines. Pharmaceutical company–developed clinical guidelines would have a low chance of being accepted as objective guidelines. The guidelines would be considered as another tool to sell more products, and their adoption by physicians would be unlikely. However, when pharmaceutical companies enter into an agreement with customers to help develop clinical guidelines, their thought leader network can be used to develop independent and objective guidelines.

Health Economic and Pharmacoeconomic Know-How

The objective of disease management is to improve the quality-cost ratio of patient care results. Therefore, the economic outcomes of interventions need to be measured. Health economics/pharmacoeconomics is a relatively young science, and there are few experts available. Due to the increasing need for economic justifications of pharmaceutical products, companies have developed extensive in-house expertise. This expertise can be used in offering services that help customers measure the value of the services performed and the medical interventions used. Additionally, the economic value of disease management programs needs to be measured.

Data Management

The development and marketing of pharmaceutical products involve the collection, analysis, and distribution of information. Pharmaceutical companies used to think of themselves as chemical companies but are now coming to realize that they are "health information management" companies. Research and development involves the gathering and analysis of information. The chemical process to produce the physical product accounts for only a small part of the effort and cost of bringing a product to market. When all the necessary information has been collected, pharmaceutical companies distribute and present the findings to health authorities like the Food and Drug Administration to seek approval for the new product. Once the product has been approved, an effective distribution of information on the product takes place. This is the key element of marketing. The extensive experience in collecting and analyzing data can be used in disease management. There are differences between managing data from tightly controlled clinical trials and managing real-life data, but most of the same tools and principles can be applied.

Medical Education and Information

The expertise in distributing information for maximum impact can be leveraged to inform and train the general public, patients, physicians, and other health care providers. Pharmaceutical companies are well respected for their ability to develop sophisticated educational materials to complement their products. These materials are used by physicians to educate their patients. Pharmaceutical companies train their personnel in house, including medical representatives, in complicated diseases and treatments. Skilled trainers and advanced training methods are available. Training and education are key components of disease management and are needed to modify the behavior of the general public, patients, and often physicians and other health care providers.

Sales Force

The sales force could take on new, or complementary, roles as educators or distributors of information that could help build and implement disease management programs. Medical representatives have good knowledge of diseases and treatments and have developed relationships with physicians. Our previous experience at Ciba (now Novartis) was that medical representatives were welcomed by physicians, and others involved in programs, in their new roles in helping to implement disease management programs. We also found that medical representatives were enthusiastic about their new role in helping to implement disease management programs.

Global Presence

All health care systems are going through some form of reform, and all systems need to reduce or maintain cost while increasing or maintaining quality of care. Therefore, all health care systems could benefit from disease management. Although disease management needs to be tailored to each unique health care system, many core principles of disease management are common across different health care systems. Players in the health care field can greatly benefit from experiences in other countries where solutions to common problems may have been found. Pharmaceutical companies, with their global presence, can help facilitate this cross-border communication.

Pharmaceutical companies are in a unique position, through their global presence, to benefit from transferring learnings from disease management programs in one country to other countries and to build cross-border and international disease management collaborations. A globally coordinated disease management approach can facilitate the development of cross-border programs. Disease management at Ciba was globally coordinated, and the company had several international programs, including pan-European programs (e.g., a comprehensive decision-support and outcomes research program in oncology), U.S.-Canadian programs (e.g., a patient training and outcomes research program for postmenopausal patients), and European-U.S. programs (e.g., a U.S.-Italian collaboration on a hypertension guidelines, training, and outcomes research program). Another example of international collaboration was a managed care organization in the United States that was about to embark on the development of clinical guidelines for epilepsy. One of our partners in the United Kingdom had already developed comprehensive guidelines. With the help of Ciba, our U.S. partner could adapt these guidelines to its needs. Our experience was that our disease management partners were enthusiastic about cross-border collaborations.

Experience in Forming and Managing Partnerships

Disease management is all about partnerships among several partners, each of whom contributes core competencies. Often, complex partnerships are necessary to achieve the best outcomes. Pharmaceutical companies have extensive experience in initiating, developing, and managing complex partnerships through research and development, copromotion, and comarketing collaborations. This professional management experience could be valuable in a disease management partnership.

KEY FACTORS FOR PHARMACEUTICAL COMPANIES' SUCCESS IN DISEASE MANAGEMENT

Disease management offers pharmaceutical companies the opportunity to build intimate relationships with their customers. To get the most out of this opportunity, there must be a full commitment from higher management. This commitment must be accompanied by financial and human resources. There must also be organizational changes to adapt to this new approach to customers, including a change in mind-set. Throughout the organization, people must shift from a "product focus" to a "customer solution focus." These customer solutions may well go beyond products. The following key factors are essential for success in disease management.

A Corporate Culture with Openness to Change, Flexibility, and Speed

To shift the thinking and practice within an organization, there must be a high degree of flexibility and an atmosphere of openness to change. The organization must also be able to react fast to adapt to changes in markets. The success of disease management is dependent on new technologies and methods of information management to ensure integration and coordination of health care components, seamless electronic communication, and management of large quantities of complex data. The development of new information technologies today is incredibly fast and could result in quick changes to the disease management landscape. Pharmaceutical companies are used to long development times and working within a market where changes occur at a slow pace. This pace is in general increasing, but in the arena of disease management and health information management (HIM), the speed of change will be incredibly high. Traditional organizational structures and decision processes in pharmaceutical companies may not be well suited to cope with this speed of change. To cope with this fast-developing field, companies may adapt their organizations and processes or keep disease management and HIM activities in separate units or organizations.

Long-Term Commitment

When entering into disease management collaborations or partnerships, the customer or partner will, to a certain degree, become dependent on the services provided by the pharmaceutical company. Pulling out of the collaboration too early could backfire and ruin a customer relationship. It is particularly important to make the commitment up front, since it is unlikely that the return on investment will be clear and measurable in the short term.

Effective Communication and Close Collaboration with Customers, Including Payers and Key Decision Makers

Pharmaceutical companies that make the commitment to disease management will need to develop new relationships with their customers that will take the form of partnerships. To do this successfully, there must be open, honest, and frequent communication. It is important for all key players who will be affected by the collaboration to be informed and comfortable with the partnership. This will include the physicians with whom the collaboration most likely will be implemented, payers, and key decision makers.

Capability for Partnerships and Alliance Management

Usually, pharmaceutical companies have experience in managing complex alliances and partnerships. It is important that the new disease management partnerships be recognized as such and that effort and resources be put into an active management of the partnership. All legal issues must be dealt with and agreed upon up front. This can be a challenge, and our experience is that it is more complex and takes longer than expected to reach agreements and to sign contracts.

Development of Interdisciplinary Teams

It is crucial to involve the necessary people in the pharmaceutical company's organization to ensure the right analysis, planning, and implementation of disease management programs. The in-house expertise that needs to be involved will come from marketing, medicine, and health or pharmacoeconomics. If disease management is left to marketing people, it will tend to become another way to communicate and build relationships with customers. If left to medical people, it will tend to become another phase IV study. If left to the health economics people, it will tend to become another economic study. High-quality disease management programs have elements of all three, but there needs to be a balance among them.

Knowledge of Diseases and Their Treatment, Outcomes, Key Cost Drivers, and Points of Intervention for Maximum Impact

It is essential to have in-depth understanding of all aspects of the diseases. Each disease must be mapped out to gain a clear understanding of how various patient groups, forms, and stages of the disease are managed. All relevant cost elements for the disease and for each intervention need to be defined to identify the key cost elements where savings can be found. Finally, elements or interventions that can be changed to improve quality of care must be identified. After a clear understanding of these elements of the disease has been established, the disease management program can be designed.

Access to Patient Information and the Ability To Integrate and Analyze the Data

Access to integrated patient data is essential for measuring the outcomes of interventions and disease management programs. The collection and evaluation of the data must be built into disease management programs. The data need to be coded so that patients cannot be identified. Another requirement is that individual physicians or physician groups be kept anonymous before the pharmaceutical company is allowed to gain access to the data. Even when neither patients nor physicians can be identified, the partner may often be reluctant to allow pharmaceutical companies access to the data. The degree of access varies from one country to another and from one partner to another. One solution may be to have a third party or a steering committee with representatives from all parties managing or taking responsibility for the data.

Alignment of Objectives and Incentives

Traditionally, objectives and incentives are not fully aligned among the "six Ps" of disease management (purchasers, patients, physicians and other health care providers, payers, policy makers, and pharmaceutical companies). For successful implementation of disease management, the incentives must be aligned among the parties involved. All parties need to work toward the objective of improving the ratio of quality of care to cost of care.

Willingness To Detach Disease Management Programs from Direct Product Sales

Customers of pharmaceutical companies tend to mistrust the industry. Frequently, companies offering disease management programs are met with suspicion, and disease management is seen as just another way to sell products. In the eyes of the customer, this suspicion tends to be confirmed when programs offered are tied directly to sales of products. A product-based approach to disease management risk gives disease management a bad name, especially when it is offered by pharmaceutical companies. Clearly, pharmaceutical companies need to gain some direct or indirect financial benefit from the programs. To overcome this problem, they may offer the customer a range of options. The customer could pay a fee for the program, share the benefits (or risks) gained from the program, or even agree to allow the company to sell more products, assuming that doing so improves clinical outcomes.

BENEFITS TO PHARMACEUTICAL COMPANIES FROM DISEASE MANAGEMENT

To offer disease management programs will require both financial and human resource investments. The return on these investments is not always obvious or immediate. The returns from pharmaceutical companies' investments in their core businesses are usually clear and can more easily be measured. To justify a continuous investment in disease management, it is important to define the expected returns. Disease management programs should be tracked to see if the expected returns materialize. The return from the investment in disease management must be quantified as much as possible but must also include returns that are less quantifiable. The benefits, or returns on disease management investments, could include the following:

- sales of disease management programs
- risk or benefit sharing
- increased sales through improved patient compliance
- formation of partnerships and interdependencies with physicians and other traditional customers
- gain in knowledge about a broader range of customer needs
- demonstration of product value through outcomes research
- building of relationships with patients
- active involvement in developing, training, and distributing clinical guidelines
- building of a positive image for the pharmaceutical company

Sales of Disease Management Programs

One obvious way to recoup investments is to charge for the programs. This could be set up as a separate profit/loss business. Another way is to use the sales to cover the cost of the programs and have the benefits come from the items below. To be able to charge for a disease management program, some beneficial outcomes (e.g., improvement of the quality-cost ratio) to the customer or partner(s) need to be demonstrated. Running a pilot program could be a way to demonstrate the improved outcomes.

Risk and Benefit Sharing

When accurate cost data can be acquired and when the disease management program has been demonstrated to reduce cost, there is an opportunity to enter into a benefit- or risk-sharing agreement. The base cost of the specific disease population needs to be measured accurately. The cost reductions from the disease management program need to be tracked over time. The arrangement could be

1. *Capitation.* The pharmaceutical company can take on the whole financial risk of a specific disease. The capitated price should include all pharmaceutical and other treatments for that disease. If the programs provided by the pharmaceutical company reduce cost, the company can keep all the savings. Conversely, the company will have to cover the excess cost if the total cost increases.
2. *Sharing of cost savings.* The pharmaceutical company can offer disease management programs for free and share the cost savings. At a predetermined and agreed-on time point (e.g., after 1 year), the cost savings can be quantified for a specific population. The savings can then be shared among

the partners involved. An example of the potential financial return from an arrangement of this kind is shown in Exhibit 8–1.

One risk of entering into risk- or benefit-sharing arrangements is that the financial returns to the pharmaceutical company will decline over time. It may be relatively easy to demonstrate cost reductions in the beginning. But if the disease management program is effective, it will become increasingly difficult to reduce cost over time, and the financial return to the pharmaceutical company from the shared benefits will decline.

Improved Patient Compliance

A clear benefit for all parties is an increase in patient compliance because it leads to the following:

- Patients take the medication as prescribed, resulting in better clinical outcomes and superior quality of care, which should lead to improved patient satisfaction.
- Physicians and payers achieve improved outcomes for their patients, resulting in more satisfied customers and reduced cost from relapses, emergency department visits, and hospitalizations.
- Pharmacists and pharmaceutical companies sell more medications.

Exhibit 8–1 Financial Returns from an Arrangement To Share Cost Savings

A study by McNabb et al[10] measured the outcomes from a group education program for children with asthma. The program cost $180 per child. The study demonstrated

- a reduction of the annual number of emergency department visits from 7.4 to 1.9 per child
- a reduction of cost by $687 per child
- a net saving of $507 per child

An equivalent saving could be demonstrated from a similar program offered by a pharmaceutical company to a customer. Assuming that the patient population was the same as above and involved 500 patients, the total savings from the program would be about $250,000. If the agreement was to split the savings equally, the pharmaceutical company would get $125,000. The total cost of the program would be $180 × 500 = $90,000. The net return would be $ 35,000, or a return on sales of 28%.

Source: Data from W.L. McNabb, et al., Self Management of Children with Asthma: AIR WISE, *American Journal of Public Health,* Vol. 75, pp. 1219–1220, © 1985.

The benefit for pharmaceutical companies can be quantified by measuring the increased sales of their product for the partner's patients.

Forming Partnerships and Interdependencies with Physicians and Other Traditional Customers

Disease management programs offered by pharmaceutical companies should complement the activities of their customers. When a pharmaceutical company has committed to a long-term relationship by offering services that improve the quality-cost ratio of patient care, the collaboration builds a partner relationship rather than a vendor relationship. It creates an interdependency between the pharmaceutical company and its customer. The disease management program will make the company more attractive to its customers and more competitive. The partnership may help build a loyalty to the pharmaceutical company. For example, Novo Nordisk, a major supplier of insulin, has no clause in its contract prohibiting its customers from using Lilly insulin. Through collaboration, Novo Nordisk has built a relationship with customers that has resulted in increased access to customers and created leverage for the company's other diabetes products.[11]

Gaining Knowledge about a Broader Range of Customer Needs

By collaborating with physicians and other customers on disease management programs, pharmaceutical companies can gain intimate knowledge about customers and their needs. This information should be used to improve R&D activities, which can be directed to respond more closely to customer needs. Access to real-life outcomes data will ensure further optimization of R&D objectives and strategies. The knowledge can also be fed back into marketing departments and can improve the effectiveness of marketing activities.

The knowledge of customers' needs can be used to develop new disease management programs in parallel with product development. The launch of disease management programs that may complement particular products can be introduced before the launch of these products to build customer intimacy and partnerships.

Demonstrating Product Value through Outcomes Research

Increasingly, pharmaceutical companies need to demonstrate the cost-effectiveness of their products to ensure inclusion in formularies and "positive lists" and exclusion from "negative lists." These data can be generated through controlled health and pharmacoeconomic studies. As more real-life data become available, pharmaceutical companies will need to demonstrate cost-effectiveness in these real-life situations. These data may, in the future, be purchased from suppliers of such data. Alternatively, pharmaceutical companies can, with their partners, generate the data themselves.

Building a Relationship with Patients and Gaining Insight into Patient Behavior

Patients are becoming increasingly involved in the treatment decision process. It therefore becomes important to build positive relationships with this customer group. Many disease management programs offered by pharmaceutical companies are directed toward patients. These programs improve outcomes of treatment, and patients' involvement is likely to improve their satisfaction. Pharmaceutical companies have the opportunity to build positive relationships with these customers. This positive relationship may help build a brand loyalty to the pharmaceutical company's products. By working closely with patients and actively eliciting feedback, pharmaceutical companies may also gain deeper insight into patient behavior that otherwise would be difficult to obtain.

Achieving Involvement in Developing, Training and Distributing Clinical Guidelines

Best-practice guidelines are increasingly becoming a part of daily practice as evidence-based medicine assumes a firmer stance (see Chapters 2 and 3). Pharmaceutical companies involved in development, distribution, and education will have limited ability to influence the guidelines themselves but can benefit indirectly. An example of how a pharmaceutical company can benefit from the distribution and training of clinical practice guidelines may be through the risk-sharing arrangements described above. Johnson & Johnson agreed to distribute and train the physicians of Group Health Cooperative of Puget Sound in the correct use of quinolones. They benefited through increased sales of their own quinolone.

Building Positive Images for Pharmaceutical Companies

By being actively involved in the improvement of total health care, pharmaceutical companies have the opportunity to improve their image. The traditional image of pharmaceutical companies can clearly be improved. Through companies' involvement in disease management and improving health care, it can easily be improved.

PHARMACEUTICAL COMPANIES' APPROACH TO DISEASE MANAGEMENT

The pharmaceutical industry has gone through a transformation from a product focus to a customer focus. It is currently moving toward a customer solutions and customer relations focus. These transformations are illustrated in Figure 8–6.

The last step toward customer solutions and relations means offering solutions beyond products to include disease management services and improved outcomes. Pharmaceutical companies have taken different strategic directions in disease management. Many companies are still in the second phase: they offer "value-added" products and services to their customers and call that disease management. The primary objective of these "value-added" products and services is, as the term implies, to add value to the pharmaceutical products with the aim of selling more products. In this case, disease management becomes another tactical marketing tool and does not constitute a move into the third phase. It is not a new strategic approach to the market. If "value-added" products and services improve the quality-cost ratio of patient care, as can be demonstrated through outcomes analysis, they may enter the realm of disease management.

Pharmaceutical companies that have truly understood the potential of disease management as a strategic new direction for the pharmaceutical industry have taken one of two general directions: building disease management internally into the existing structures or creating external units or organizations, as illustrated in Figure 8–7.

Several companies are at various stages in the process of moving into phase 3. These include (name of the disease management unit in parentheses) Lilly (Inte-

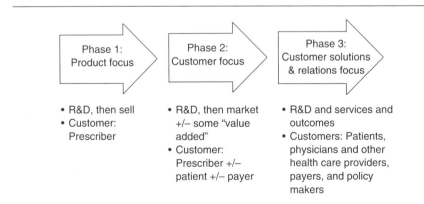

Figure 8–6 Evolution of Pharmaceutical Companies' Strategic Focus

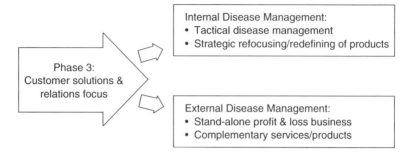

Figure 8–7 Disease Management in Pharmaceutical Companies

---

grated Disease Management), SmithKline Beecham (SB Healthcare Services), Novartis (formerly Ciba and Sardoz), Zeneca (Stuart Disease Management), Novo Nordisk, Bristol-Myers Squibb, Merck, Glaxo, Pfizer (Pfizer Healthcare Systems), and Pharmacia & Upjohn (Greenstone Healthcare Solutions). Examples of the different directions they have taken are

- internal disease management with a strategic refocus and redefined products (eg, Novo Nordisk)
- external disease management with stand-alone profit-and-loss organizations (eg, Stuart Disease Management, owned by Zeneca)
- external disease management offering complementary services and products (eg, SmithKline Beecham)[12]

All these companies are beginning to offer a range of disease management and information management services. In spite of the uncertainties of the return on their investments, they have taken the lead in the industry. If this strategy turns out to be the strategy for the future, they will have an advantage in the future marketplace over companies that have not yet made this strategic decision.

Three pharmaceutical companies acquired pharmacy benefit managers (PBMs) in 1993 and 1994: Merck (Medco for $6.6 billion), Lilly (PCS for $4.1 billion), and SmithKline Beechham (Diversified for $2.3 billion). One of the key reasons for acquiring these PBMs was to control the distribution channel and increase the parent company's share of drugs sold through the PBM. However, regulators placed restrictions on the companies' ability to influence the PBMs to increase their parents' share. The results have been mixed. Lilly's share of prescriptions in PCS declined by 6.9% in the first half of 1996, while its share increased by 7.2% in all 87 PBMs surveyed by IMS. At the time of this writing, Lilly had just written down its PCS investment by over $2 billion. SmithKline Beecham's share of prescriptions in Diversified increased by 16% in the first half of 1996. However, during the same time period, Lilly's share of prescriptions in Diversified increased by 19%, and Merck's share increased by 32%. Merck has done better with its PBM. Its share in Medco increased by 32%, while Merck's share in the remaining PBMs increased by 20%.[13]

However, these three companies have stated that they acquired PBMs not only to increase the parent company's share but to develop and offer sophisticated services to their managed-care customers.[14] The head of SB Healthcare Services, T. Yamada, stated that "Diversified will allow SB to be involved in the whole business of healthcare solutions above and beyond simply providing pills."[14] PCS offers a range of disease management programs and has boosted its outcomes research department from two people in 1995 to 11 in 1996 to meet its customers needs.[14] PBMs are already in the service business and have well-established relationships with managed care organizations. PBMs can build on their current activities and strengths to develop disease management programs, which may include

- integrating their pharmaceutical data with clinical and nonpharmaceutical cost data (which would require close cooperation and sharing of data with managed care organizations)
- monitoring patient compliance through monitoring of prescription refills
- helping develop, monitor, and enforce prescribers' compliance with treatment guidelines
- providing information technology and information management skills

Combining these strengths with the strengths of the parent companies could give Merck, Lilly, and SmithKline Beecham competitive advantages. Several other pharmaceutical companies have realized the advantages of working with PBMs and have formed various types of alliances with PBMs (e.g. Pfizer, Johnson & Johnson, and Sardoz with Value Rx).

FUTURE OF DISEASE MANAGEMENT IN THE PHARMACEUTICAL INDUSTRY

Physicians and other customers of pharmaceutical companies are rapidly becoming very sophisticated and are demanding more than just effective and safe products. They are increasingly demanding solutions to their health care problems, whether these are pharmaceutical or other products, services, or other offerings that achieve the objective of improving the quality-cost ratio of patient care. This transformation of markets is still in its early stages. It is sometimes useful to examine how other companies have managed to transform themselves to respond to new demands from their customers. One example of a company that has undergone a successful transformation is Xerox Corporation. This company was previously in the photocopying machine industry. They were competing with other companies offering very similar products. The leading companies in the industry would offer the best photocopying machines or the best price. The industry then realized that customers also made their choice of photocopying machines based on another dimension: service. The companies would offer services to ensure that the customer's photocopying machine worked. Should the machine break down, the service person would be there within a short time to fix it. This became increasingly important, since there were no major differentiating features among the machines. Customers were dependent on having fully functioning photocopying machines. The added services were a kind of "value-added" service, but the companies were still selling photocopying machines.

Xerox then realized that customers needed not only photocopying machines but effective ways of managing their documents. Xerox underwent a transformation and redefined its business from producing photocopying machines to offering customer solutions: *document management.* This meant a redirection of the whole company, including R&D. Xerox would still offer photocopying machines, but as a part of a wider product and service package. This package would include other pieces of hardware like computers, various kinds of software necessary for management of documents, various services, and consulting. Xerox explored which types of documents their customers needed to manage and offered solutions concerning how best to manage them. One such document was a registration package for a new pharmaceutical product that had to be submitted to health authorities. This package contained a huge number of documents that had to be presented in the best possible way to improve the chances for achieving the marketing approval. Xerox would offer a complete package to manage the documents. Xerox would even offer services enabling electronic submission of the registration dossier, which would mean that photocopying machines would not be necessary at all. Xerox has been highly successful in transforming itself and is now promoting itself as "the Document Company."

Another company that is undergoing a transition from a product focus to an integrated product and service focus is General Electric (GE). Jack Welch, GE's chairman, has created the most valuable company in the world, with a total market capitalization of $200 billion. Mr. Welch is again remaking his company, this time to change the industrial units of GE to take a bigger share of related services, building on GE's core industrial strengths. This move has been undertaken both to expand the business to include services and to build broader relationships with customers. The reengineering guru Michael Hammer sees GE as a bellwether: "This is the next big wave in American industry; the product you sell is only one component of your business."[15]

Prospectus

Is the health care market forcing the pharmaceutical industry to transform itself from providing pills to providing solutions? Will pharmaceutical companies be able to compete on the efficacy, safety, and quality of their products alone in the future? The industry has already experienced that marketing a "me-too" product is becoming increasingly difficult and costly and may not be a profitable option. Breakthrough products will still be a profitable business in the future. It is, however, becoming increasingly difficult to find and develop breakthrough products. Alternative formulas for success must be found.

Pharmaceutical companies have in reality already transformed themselves from pharmaceutical manufacturers, or chemical drug companies, to managers of information. An examination of the cost structures in pharmaceutical companies today reveals that only a small portion of total cost comes from chemical synthesis and production. The largest portion of R&D cost by far is the generation and management of information. Successful marketing is effectively distributing information and building strong relationships with customers. If pharmaceutical companies, in reality, are sophisticated managers of health-related information and customer relationships, the transformation to becoming sophisticated "disease managers" should be a relatively small step.

Should pharmaceutical companies abandon their core business of pharmaceutical products? It would probably not be a good idea, but it is crucial for success that they reexamine the business they are in and redefine the products and services they offer. This process must be undertaken *now* since the leaders in the pharmaceutical industry in the next century will be determined today. The companies that are able to transform their business today will be among the winners in the next century. As Abraham Lincoln once said, "We must plan for the future, because people who stay in the present will remain in the past."

References

1. Soumerai SB, et al. Effects of Medicaid drug-payment limits on admission to hospitals and nursing homes. *N Engl J Med.* 1991;325:1072–1077.
2. Broshy B, Kemeny CR, Nesbitt A, Wurster TS. Managing for a wired health care industry. *In Vivo.* July/August 1996;8–14.
3. Felton T, Lister G. Coopers & Lybrand; 1996.
4. Chataway M. The information highway: route statistics. Presented at "The Strategic Use of the Internet in the Pharmaceutical Industry"; February 26–27, 1996; London, England.
5. *E-Med News.* March 12, 1996:11.
6. Morrison I. *The Second Curve: Managing the Velocity of Change.* New York, NY: Ballantine Books; 1996.

7. Eli Lilly launches new approach to health care. *News Edge*. March 27, 1996.

8. Todd WE. A partnership model for asthma disease management. National Jewish Center, Denver Colorado. Presented at Disease Management IIR Conference; January 25–27, 1995; Philadelphia, Pennsylvania.

9. Bartlett E. Cost-benefit analysis of patient education: new trends in patient education. In: *Proceedings from Patient Education 2000*. Geneva, Switzerland: Elsevier Science; 1995:87–91.

10. McNabb WL, et al. Self management of children with asthma: AIR WISE. *Am J Public Health*. 1985;75:1219–1220.

11. Cassak D. Novo Nordisk and the challenge of disease management. *In Vivo*. May 1996:41–52.

12. Pigache P. Name of the game: interview with Bishop, H., Head of SB Healthcare Services. *Pharmaceutical Visions*. February 1996:62–66.

13. IMS America Ltd. purchases of drug managers are questioned. *Wall Street J*. November 20, 1996.

14. Purchase of drug managers are questioned. *Wall Street J*. November 20, 1996.

15. Jack Welch's encore. *Bus Week*. October 28, 1996:42–50.

CHAPTER 9

Disease Management Purchasers' Perspectives

Larry L. Hipp

Health care in this country has evolved from a cottage industry to an industry of rapidly changing organizational entities responding to the economic impact of rising health care costs. Public and private purchasers of health care have shown great agility in tossing the cost-shifting ball back and forth into each other's court. The history of this evolution is well described by Couch and Warshaw.[1] They outline the economic, social, and political forces that have converged to accelerate the profound changes seen now. As they predicted, American industry has taken the challenge and been the real driver in applying the lessons learned in continuous quality improvement to the health care industry.

The private purchaser initiatives have been multifaceted, as American industry itself tends to be spanning a continuum of very small to very large enterprises. An early industry leader in requiring quality initiatives of suppliers was the Xerox Corporation. Other large purchasers have defined their own expectations for quality care reflective of their own corporate culture and needs.

Health care, affected as it is by social, cultural, and economic forces, necessarily remains a local phenomenon in this country. For this reason, there has been a rapid development of community-based purchasing alliances formed by local companies, large and small, as well as by national companies in concert with them on a local level. These will be more substantially discussed later in the chapter. In addition, national companies have banded together to maximize their purchasing influence in local communities. As will be seen, these purchasing coalitions have exerted and are exerting the single most influential impact on the quest for quality health services. They wish to improve health and productivity in their work force. Couch and Warshaw write that "although not many companies are currently [i.e., in 1991] directly contracting with health care suppliers, it is predicted that large companies and multiple-employer trusts will be contracting directly with plans by the end of this century."[1(p 387)] As we will see, coalitions have begun contracting with plans, and in at least one, contracting is beginning with providers themselves. The richness of the private marketplace allows for the diversity of these initiatives and thus the trial of many approaches simultaneously.

American industry is in an increasingly competitive international marketplace that requires continuous improvement in quality and cost of products. The move to incorporate this value equation into the total health supplier community is forcing a shift from selecting simple, low-cost supplier options to placing emphasis on cost and quality. These new approaches require refinement of processes and improved outcomes that are now present to a larger extent in contracts with health providers. Population size and data collection are key elements in efforts to substantiate improvement. For this reason, disease management is and will be of more and more interest to providers and purchasers, since it is a population-based activity substantiating the value equation.

PURCHASERS' PERSPECTIVES

The increasing emphasis on quality and disease management has forced the purchasing community to recognize a demand for skill and knowledge sets not heretofore present. In most cases, the benefits community has had to learn to communicate expectations and get closer to the professional medical community for quality results. Likewise, occupationally trained physicians are in some cases being asked by employers and benefits colleagues to play a larger role in the selection and monitoring of quality measurements for suppliers. In a positive way, this has forged a link between traditional employee-based, prevention-focused occupational health programs and the overall health of employees and dependents.

Many in the private purchasing world, specifically in occupational health programs, will say, "Disease management? We've been doing this for a long time." Over the years, a range of activities, programs, and approaches to managing acute and chronic illnesses in the workplace have captured the attention of the occupational physician. Most proposed solutions have shared the stated purpose of increasing worker productivity in a workplace interested in its employees' health and well-being. The programs tend to wax and wane depending on evaluations of efficacy, cost efficiency, business focus, organization, and other vagaries of the workplace at any given time. The redefinition of the term *disease management* is a product of the evolution of the managed care market. The various stakeholders have seen the need and opportunity to address the core issue of changing how health and illness are managed.

So what makes the "new" disease management different from these former programs? Coined by the pharmaceutical industry in the early 1990s, the term *disease management* refers to activities done under various rubrics with new and important characteristics that set it apart. Competing definitions are abundant in the literature and language of the marketplace. Scott MacStravic differentiates management from marketing by target population.[2] He points out that management gives its attention primarily to internal targets: employees, medical staff, and suppliers. Marketing, in contrast, focuses almost exclusively on customers, external targets that have grown to include employers and insurers as well as patients. Disease management, in his lexicon, addresses consumers as the primary focus.

A recent article by Kozma et al[3] presents an excellent conceptual view of how outcomes research and disease management are brought together to provide efficient care of populations. Figure 9–1 schematically depicts the process.

Kozma et al cogently point out potential conflicts brought about by maximizing the care of the health of individuals as opposed to the health of populations. One such conflict is that between prescriber autonomy and the guidance provided by disease management programs. Another is the conflict between cost and quality, which may result in situations where significantly reducing costs and managing disease at the highest quality level are not compatible. Last but not least to the purchasing world is the conflict of interests among stakeholders in the process, including patients, providers, producers, and payers, as well as insurers, pharmaceutical companies, pharmacy benefit management companies, provider organizations, individual providers, private companies, academic institutions, and patient organizations. The need to factor stakeholders' interests into any disease management program is vital.

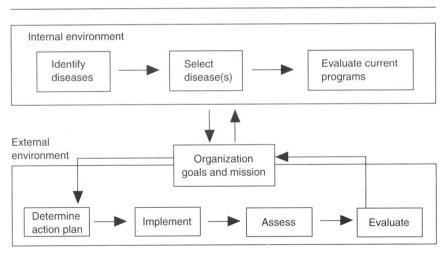

Figure 9–1 Process of Disease State Management. *Source:* Reprinted with permission from C.M. Kozma, K.A. Kaa, and C.E. Reeder, A Model for Comprehensive Disease State Management, The Journal of Outcomes Management, Vol. 4, No. 1, p. 7, © 1997.

In the context of this chapter, I will rely upon a commonly expressed definition of disease management as a process-driven, defined-population–based approach that identifies an at-risk disease-specific group.[4] Examples of populations are asthma patients in an asthma management program for all beneficiaries of a specific company, or all covered lives in a managed care plan. Interventions are well-defined medical and psychosocially described programs of care that measure clinical as well as other outcomes of this care, such as rapid return to function, increased ability to self-manage the disease, and a better quality of life. The most distinctive feature of disease management is that it is an information-driven approach that can measure more than just single-encounter–based clinical episodes. By applying process- and information-based algorithms, it allows for process and clinical changes in the patient in a dynamic, fluid, and quality-driven manner. It encompasses behavioral and clinical measurements broader in scope than other historical methodologies. Disease management offers the possibility of effecting changes in worker productivity through collaborative interventions that join classical in-house medical programs to health and benefit programs for employees and their families. It can be a bridge between traditional separations of health responsibilities for internal occupational medical programs and for general employee health benefits. Physicians can see expanded opportuntities for improving health outcomes while continuously learning how to improve treatments to achieve optimal health status improvements.

This chapter will primarily focus on disease management interests in the private sector, that is, the commercial market. This contrasts with but does not exclude the governmental agencies responsible for mandating the delivery of health services to the population. However, the interests are quite the same in the public sector for those professionals involved in maintaining the health of employees in the workplace. For as a health care system takes shape under private health care reform, the interests of the public sector become closer to those of private purchasers. The auto industry, led by General Motors, has initiated what it is calling a "community approach" toward curbing health care costs. Being unable because of labor considerations to change the very rich, almost "first-dollar" coverage for care, the company has developed strategies that have allowed it to identify communities in which there are high worker populations and to compare cost and utilization data with those for other areas of the country. In so doing, it is now focusing on communities with high cost and utilization and introducing multifaceted approaches toward implementing change. In one of the communities, one of the hospital systems is moving to close four hospitals and consolidate into a single medical center. Also as a result of this initiative, the company has reduced job classifications in the patient-related area from 250 to 3. This represents a radical change in the relationship of the public and private sectors. The primary emphasis has been on influencing the caregivers in the community. Physicians are encouraged to be partners in this health-focused initiative.

Some skeptics suggest that there also must be some curbing of employees' use of and demand on the system for long-lasting change. The basic strategy of the automakers has been to deal with health suppliers much as they have dealt with parts suppliers, by setting quality and cost standards to qualify for their business. Although this may not be a universal model, it works well in communities where the automakers exhibit significant financial influence and has elements of application in many settings.[5,6] The influence of federal, state, and local governments in the quality of care will be significant as they move more toward offering health services or placing populations in managed care. They are beginning to initiate more quality demands as they contract with managed care organizations. This ultimately leads to focus on and intervention in diseases that are high cost, high frequency, and susceptible to preventive initiatives. It is clear, however, that the influence of the government as the largest single purchaser of health care will be substantial in bringing private and public interests closer together. The impact of managed care plans for Medicaid and Medicare recipients is already resulting in substantial changes in health care delivery.

The literature does not abound with substantive articles on purchasers and their interest and successes in disease management. Much of the work to date has been done in proprietary organizations, and the arrangements have been in place for too short a time to measure the long-term effects. To the extent that available information allows, I will describe activities in traditional occupational health programs, provide examples of new initiatives in disease management, and discuss some barriers, opportunities, and implications for the future.

OCCUPATIONAL AND ENVIRONMENTAL MEDICINE PERSPECTIVE

Several major health-realted activities have dimensions in common with disease management. Occupational medical programs in particular have engaged in various aspects of health management for decades. Their services have ranged from full management of employees' and their families' health problems with on-site medical facilities to a more recent trend focusing primarily on services and interventions that are directed toward the environmental stressors in the workplace and their health impact on workers. The range of programs is as diverse as the business community that has supported them. With the advent of interventions for lifestyle changes such as fitness, smoking cessation, and health promotion that are directed toward the "healthy" work force, the role of occupational health programs has seen some "out-of-the-walls" expansion. Opportunities have been provided to workers' families and dependents. These programs are population based and are substantially lifestyle change opportunities. Though altruistically motivated in some instances, the programs are generally driven by data of various types demonstrating an increase in worker productivity. Interventions such as fitness, nutrition, smoking cessation, and stress reduction show positive outcomes. This population-based approach, with its educational component, provides a foundation for, and bridge for expansion to, the more traditional episodic clinical interventions prevalent in the occupational medical world. Although there have been and continue to be challenges to the efficiency and cost-effectiveness of these programs, they have set a model before the purchasing community that lends itself to disease management (population based, information driven). The physician has developed more tools to demonstrate value-added health programs to company management.

For decades, occupational health programs have been involved in the management of workers' compensation illnesses and injuries—that is, those health problems arising by legal definition in and/or out of the course of employment. In many cases, very sophisticated case management programs have evolved. They are different from disease management as currently defined, however, because they have been directed at episodic care related to the specific compensable illness or injury episode. Even more significantly, they have been individually focused as a case management exercise. The demarcation between work-related illness and concurrent "noncompensable" illnesses has been required to be distinct, often for legal purposes. However, attempts toward defining causation in the workers' compensation environment involve epidemiological approaches similar to those used in disease management. Assessing environmental aspects related to the development or occurrence of disease or injury has required introducing psychosocial variables that make the occupational physician comfortable in evaluating the whole patient. The complex relationship between entities managing a patient under workers' compensation guidelines today collides with the managed care networks and their defined provider populations. It is in the interest of workers' compensation programs and managed care networks to become more congruent with disease management programs. This at some level is being approached by the integration both of these artificially defined management exercises into single networks.

In January 1997, a seminar entitled "Financial Integration of Workers' Compensation, Group Health and Disability" was held at the National Workers' Compensation Institute in San Diego. Although the title would indicate that only financial issues were presented, a variety of methodologies described involved sophisticated information gathering to identify high-risk illness events, rationales for the savings resulting from an integrated program, and strategic goal-setting models for making decisions about risk sharing. The models for consideration included integrating workers' compensation with managed care plans, as well as integrating disability, workers' compensation, and managed care plans for all employees. It was shown that savings result from combined administration, reductions in cash outlays by monthly premium payments, lower stop-loss premiums as a result of integration, reduced litigation expense through provision of similar benefits on and off the job, and management of medical and disability claims for occupational and nonoccupational events. Barriers to effective implementation include enabling legislation to account for interstate programs for national corporations, tax implications, and the conflict between life, health, property, and casualty insurance areas. Establishing teams to implement such programs effectively requires coordination of a stakeholder list much larger than that in the usual managed care arena.

Corporations that have elected to manage short- and long-term disability programs have established medical case management programs internally that provide acute and chronic disease management. Though directed at encouraging appropriate medical services to employees that result in early return to function, the primary motivator has been reducing absenteeism. Hence, these programs have not engaged the families of those workers or the retiree population. The interventions are related only to the acute episode resulting in an absence from work. Return to employment generally signals the end of the intervention. The experience in case management with this population could offer an easy expansion to a broader base of disease management interventions. The data from this activity are clearly a valuable addition to a database that integrates disease management and functional capacity. Guidelines adopted for managing disability programs need to be integrated into any disease management effort. They are complementary and lead hopefully to increased functional capacity and thus worker productivity, a win-win situation for all parties.

The 1970s and 1980s heralded the introduction of formalized management of chronic disease in the workplace, again limited to those actively at work. With the advent at the time of a new generation of more effective treatment agents, the most popular program was the treatment of hypertension. The treatments were driven by well-defined protocols but were never broadly introduced. Relationships between the treatment regimen and the role of the private treating physician, as well as resource and cost-effectiveness issues, were barriers to broad incorporation in the occupational environment. These were perhaps the first efforts in the purchaser's workplace that addressed management of single disease entities within a defined population that included pharmaceutical administration regimens.

HEALTH PROMOTION AND DEMAND MANAGEMENT

Health promotion programs paradoxically have set a tone for the introduction of disease management concepts. They require elements of data collection, population approaches, and evaluation that have allowed the purchasing community to view the health of the working population in that different context. Although there is much value in these programs in the workplace, the difficulty in demonstrating to management their immediate value in a cost-driven atmosphere continues to be a struggle. Concurrent with the advent of managed care was the introduction of the concept of demand management in the health promotion literature and services. A shift from health promotion and a primary intervention strategy in the workplace to a strategy of demand management that embodies self-care has occurred swiftly. Traditional health promotion firms now include a range of services and programs that apply intervention strategies refined in health promotion to disease management processes. Telephone services offering self-care decision algorithms, healthy lifestyle actions, management of illness episodes, and specific disease management strategies are available and are promoted under the banner of health promotion. These vendors have been very aggressive in the purchasing marketplace.

To give an idea of the magnitude and diversity of offerings, two of these vendors offer such services as

- health assessments and self-management programs for low-risk and high-risk populations
- a call center system for inbound and outbound calls to high-risk populations that can be carved into a case management program or outsourced to them
- an administrative module
- evidence-based decision-support tools for physicians to assist them in determining best practices and treatment pathways at the point of treatment
- health assessment instruments to identify accurately and confidentially the 20% of participants within a population who would consume 50% of the health care dollars spent in the subsequent 12 to 18 months
- skill training about the disease and about support services
- behavior modification programs
- educational materials
- continuing medical education programs
- informational mailings and newsletters
- disease-specific mailings

This is only a partial list of the services offered by these organizations to providers, payers, and health plans. (N.R. Richardson, Preferred Health Systems, LLC, written communication, January 1997; D. Soutendijk, Performance Health, personal communication, 1997).

In his article "The Total Quality Revolution," Couch describes the evolution of American industry from the vertical model to the quality model driven by information management and attention to internal as well as external customers:

The central dilemma, then, for benefits managers concerns how to keep their organizations' internal customers healthy, happy, and productive while simultaneously pleasing their chief financial officers. Likewise the insurance companies must transform themselves into information management agencies with the health benefits managers as their counterparts and strategic partners in helping collect, analyze, and make available in useful reports information to permit these stakeholders to optimize their health and that of their dependents in the following ways:

1. By obtaining the information necessary from employers to perform health status or needs assessments of employee populations at particular points in their lives;

2. By assembling and matching with these employee populations the optimal mix of primary and specialty physicians, in-patient and out-patient facilities, and ancillary services;

3. By evaluating the utilization of these employees of the health care delivery systems and correlating this utilization with clinical outcomes, improved productivity and satisfaction, fewer workdays lost, and costs saved at various critical junctures in the course of the partnership between employer and health insurer;

4. By demonstrating the value added to the employers and their workforces in improving employers' ability to meet and exceed their internal customers' needs and expectations for superior value health programs; and

5. By being able to demonstrate that this type of partnership model adds greater value to companies' competitiveness and productivity through the improved health status and satisfaction of these companies' workforces than have more traditional managed care systems.[7]

Couch suggests that for health care "value" purchasing, there need to be definitions of provider quality and cost-effectiveness, systems for measuring, standards, criteria for provider selection, and methods to establish and continually adjust provider reimbursement levels on the basis of the demonstrated value of provider services.

Relationships between the physician managers of occupational health programs and the benefits managers purchasing health programs for employees vary, but in general they have not been too close. The strongest ties between occupational physicians and benefits managers have been in the management of worker's compensation because of the close relationship between the need for authorization of payments to meet state statutes relevant to process and medical care rendered pusuant to the law. The advent of managed care has resulted in a rapidly changing environment requiring redefinition of roles and establishment of new partnerships in the benefits-purchasing world. Benefits managers have found themselves confronted with issues in quality of care in selecting health plans that were heretofore nonexistent. In some cases, physician managers of occupational medical programs have found themselves with new opportunities for input into the selection of health benefits plans. The total quality management (TQM) approach that most purchasers have had to take with these vendors has required expertise in clinical areas that in many cases has not been available. In some cases, physicians have assumed the full responsibility for health care plans as well as internal medical programs. Benefits managers have been approached by vendors offering a bewildering array of services. Vendors offer carve-outs for managing pharmaceutical, mental health, and disease-specific entities, as well as others. The occupational physician in some cases has become the partner in evaluating the medical quality aspects of these plans.

Another source widely used for assistance in selection by purchasers is the consulting firm. In addition to their benefits expertise, consulting firms have engaged physicians with insight into management aspects and an understanding of utilization and quality-of-care elements. In this manner, consulting firms have become a strong influence on purchasing benefits managers. Collaboration between the consultant, occupational physicians, and benefit managers has been instrumental in shaping purchasers' expectations for quality-of-care initiatives in health plans.

THE PURCHASING COMMUNITY

The purchasing community is hardly a homogeneous group. Given that businesses that employ 1000 or more workers make up only about 20% of the work force, there is a wide array of types of businesses and needs for health services. The reality is that by their market influence, the large employers may exert heavy influence on products and services in the health marketplace. The transition of the health care marketplace since the demise of governmental health care reform has been significantly driven by these large employers and the emergence of coalitions of employers of varying sizes. The coalitions engage in the business of developing purchasing activities, measurement objectives, and community efforts leveraged by their market influence. In many communities, these coalitions account for large percentages of the covered lives. In some cases, they have included providers to develop collaborative efforts in achieving their purposes. Though often competitors in business, coalition members have found a common purpose in trying to improve health care delivery.

The coalitions continue to increase in number and offer the small as well as the larger employers a voice for their needs. Sean Sullivan, president and chief executive officer of the National Business Coalition on Health, a Washington group that monitors and advises coalitions, has effectively described the goals and evolution of these coalitions in many forums.[8] He details how purchasers are moving along the value curve from price discounting, to cost reduction, to quality improvement, to value enhancement. They are looking at trends—long- and short-term integration, capitation, contracting arrangements, management of outcomes instead of costs, and ultimately letting consumers choose. Arrangements in the coalitions include partnerships with physicians and other providers, consumer cooperatives, and other stakeholders. Quality improvements include measures to improve efficiency, practice guidelines, and outcomes measurements.

The growth of purchasing coalitions speaks to the influence they exert on the marketplace. As of 1995, they represented more than 30 million covered lives of employees and dependents of 8000 businesses.[9] Though all groups do not actually collectively purchase health care, they effectively prod providers and plans to cut prices and improve performance. The growth of the coalitions is shown in Figure 9–2.

In Minnesota, the Buyers Health Care Action Group, which is composed of 23 employers and now state employee health purchasers, has effected considerable change in the health care market. It was so successful in leveraging cost reductions that the number of competitors in the market coalesced to just a couple of dominant players. Consequently, the ability to leverage price reductions diminished. The new direction taken by this coalition is to bypass the big organizers of health care and purchase directly. The purchasing group has been very effective in taking out the savings, but the real challenge is in producing long-term changes in the

---

Gaining Strength in Numbers

The National Business Coalition on Health doubled its membership between 1992 and 1995 as new regional coalitions were formed and more employers joined existing coalitions.

Number of coalitions	Year	Number of employers represented
46	1992	4,000
60	1993	5,550
73	1994	6,725
90	1995	8,000

Figure 9–2 Growth in Health Care Purchasing Coalitions, 1992–1995. *Source:* Copyright Business & Health, made possible by a professional grant from Hoechst Marion Roussel.

health care system. The coalition is also contracting for methodologies and services to continue the drive for quality improvement in the health care suppliers. They believe this will lead to better health outcomes for their employees. More attention to the issue of health care quality will be provided later in the chapter. The ultimate health outcome depends on the ability of the plans and providers to show that they have initiated and measured improvement in the health of the population that they serve, whether by preventive initiatives, disease management, or reduction in demand by the population.

Another example of a specific community initiative is the Memphis Business Group on Health, which was formed in 1985 to act as a purchasing group and collective quality-setting organization. In the first year, they had only one bid for services, but today they routinely obtain 20% discounts from their hospitals. They also run their own case management and utilization review services, another twist in the differences seen in local markets.

Cleveland Health Quality Choice (CHQC) is a collaborative partnership between business, hospitals, and physicians designed to share information about health care quality among the five founding groups: the Greater Cleveland Hospital Association, representing local hospitals; the Academy of Medicine, representing 2900 area physicians; Cleveland Tomorrow, an organization of corporate chief executive officers, whose mission is to make Cleveland a more competitive and attractive environment for business; the Health Action Council of Northeast Ohio; and the Council of Smaller Enterprises, an organization of 12,900 smaller businesses that has recently received national attention as a model for group health care purchasing. The model is described well by Sirio and Harper.[10] The resulting data are shared in a public report that is available through retail outlets such as pharmacies in a less detailed format. It is a good example of disparate groups of stakeholders developing information to show improvement in the areas examined. The successful methodology includes

- rigorous examination of the validity and reliability of the risk adjustment tools
- a commitment to refine and update a process of data collection, analysis, and reporting that allows hospital administrator and physician feedback
- an external audit process for hospital data to ensure data integrity
- open discussions about the most appropriate methods to report data
- timely reporting of current data
- a well planned start-up and testing period with adequate time for the provider community to examine the results before widespread and public dissemination

Among the more aggressive coalitions has been the Pacific Business Group on Health in California. The coalition, which consists of 30 major California employers (23 of them in the purchasing group), embarked on a collective negotiation strategy in 1993.[9] They first established to identify objective criteria for comparison of providers and plans, ranging from price to quality issues. They found little reason for the variation in charges being experienced by various employers for populations with similar risks. Subsequent collective negotiating resulted in major savings in premiums and administrative costs, the latter accomplished by standardizing benefit structures for the whole group. The coalition has included in its purchasing requirements stringent medical quality standards.

The Massachusetts Health Care Purchasing Group (MHCPG) is a Boston-based group that does not engage in collective purchasing and includes private and public employers as well as the state's Medicaid program. It accomplishes its goal by setting target percentage rate increases that its participating members expect participating health maintenance organizations (HMOs) to meet. It describes a ripple effect among noncoalition members, who are often offered rate reductions simply to keep them from joining.

Coalitions are market specific and are all quite different because no two markets are alike. This poses something of a dilemma for the multistate employers whose benefit managers wish to keep the benefits consistent for their employees. Those coalitions that have represented employees are often bound by national labor contracts to provide the same benefits to all of their constituencies. The National HMO Purchasing Coalition, founded in 1995, enables employers to negotiate and purchase health care in 27 markets collectively. The group consists of 10 multistate employers, including American Express, IBM, Merrill Lynch, and Sears, representing more than 600,000 covered lives. One of the real challenges the group faced was agreeing on a standard HMO benefit, which they did accomplish. They then agreed on a common methodology to evaluate HMOs in the 27 markets. They used quality methodology, including chart reviews with all of the HMOs. According to Lou Ann Cash, director of compensation and benefits for American Express, the goal was to examine the management of the very sick enrollee in these plans.[9] The group reports very significant savings to its corporations as a result of this initiative and continues to look at additional ways to accomplish its goal of value-based quality services. It is committed to the latter because it is aware that only in that arena will it fully accomplish its objectives.[11]

Not all efforts by coalitions achieve what they initially set out to do. The Cincinnati Payor Initiative was a group of four companies in the Cincinnati area that collaborated with hospitals and a health care data consulting firm to get more information about the health care options available in their community.[12] This was a 3-year initiative that was to result in the selection of the best performing hospitals by the initiative. Actually, the results were reported as astounding after the first measurement year in 1992. The data were clearly used by the institutions for improving their performance. However, for a variety of reasons, the collaborating corporations have not yet used the data for selection purposes. Though not ongoing, the effort did raise a new level of awareness of cost-quality considerations to bring about payer involvement.

There has been a slow but growing recognition by providers that the early successes in controlling costs with managed care have been driven by limiting access and discounting fees from providers. Though the promise of managed care was reduced cost and improved quality, the deliverable was and still remains in large part the management of costs and access. This is not consistent with a total quality approach and results in short-term successes, as purchasers know. Fallout from this has been manifested by strong outcries from employee, union, and governmental interests. They have objected to limited stays in hospitals for certain conditions, such as pregnancy and coronary bypass procedures. They have complained about too severe restrictions of providers in the community. They do not like the gatekeeper concept. The purchasing community has no desire to alienate these interests. They are not interested in having the government intervene, as it recently has in mandating specific requirements for coverage in health plans, such as, lengths of stay for deliveries. They prefer not to alienate the unions or incur work stoppages based on cost sharing if there are other acceptable solutions to the problem of costs. The balance between cost and quality remains a moving target.

The purchasing community during its drive toward a reduction in escalating health costs has seen its own organizational and business focus change. More and more organizations, in their reengineering efforts toward a TQM approach to doing business, focus on increasing the employee's involvement in the decision process. Ultimately, this allows them to make health decisions better and take an active part in the selection of plans suitable to their individual purposes. With purchaser expectation of cost reduction with improved quality, accountability rests within the plans themselves. Disease management, the mantra of the managed care industry at the moment, is a concept of which many purchasers are aware. But many feel that the responsibility for implementing this rests within plans. Although employers are viewed as a target in marketing for disease management, they have had varying experience with direct contact from vendors. It is not that employers specifically want disease management. What they want is lower costs.[13] As one examines recent health management newsletters, it is clear that most disease management marketing efforts are being directed toward the providers and managed care organizations.[14,15] This is consistent with many purchasers' attitudes.

Disease management is a population-based approach that is information driven. Large employers have large databases that contain information collected internally as well as from various contracted vendors such as pharmacy plans, health insurance plans, workers' compensation plans, short- and long-term disability plans, and, in some cases, health promotion activities. These data can be a valuable resource in identifying target populations in collaboration with their partners. The ability to translate the data into useful information, however, is generally resource and skill limited within the business world. Large employers often can forge partnerships with disease management vendors and others to use these data successfully for targeting disease management interventions. Smaller companies may be able to pool data through their vendors. However, a challenge to the utilization of this data in targeting populations is the potential sensitivity and ethical consideration of identifying individuals in the purchaser population for intervention. Any disease management program that hints of coercion, negative incentives, or other negative outcomes will be challenged by management and union interests. The right to confidentiality, the unwillingness to reveal certain health information to employers, and the ability to make choices about compliance with certain treatment regimens are important issues. They need to be examined in the process of data sharing. Purchasers and, where applicable, their union representatives will wish to examine them very carefully.

The total quality approach requires changes in processes and basic approaches in the way work is done. Though the purchasing community is and will be requiring ongoing cost reductions, it is looking for the health industry to provide these methodologies. Disease management is one of the strategies that the purchasing world is looking at carefully and embracing with various levels of enthusiasm. Various approaches to incorporate the disease management process are the name of the game in the purchasing community. With these influences in mind, a variety of approaches by purchasers have already developed and will subsequently be described.

THE ACCREDITATION AND MEASUREMENT COMMUNITY

In their initial efforts to reduce the escalating costs for health services, purchasers have not been oblivious to the impact on service to their employee populations. It does not behoove them to purchase new products that result in poor health results, loss of productivity, and internal complaints from their employees. They are accustomed to placing requirements on vendors for financial objectives as well as quality objectives. However, with the advent of the new multifaceted organizations developed by the providers and insurers, the business community has found itself in the position of not having knowledge of the kinds of measures or outcomes that would provide comparative information among suppliers. It has tended to look to third-party independent organizations to set levels and monitor the performance of suppliers. There has long been a well-accepted accreditation organization for hospitals. The Joint Commission on Accreditation of Healthcare Organizations (hereafter referred to as "Joint Commission") has set the "gold standard" for hospitals throughout the country. With the advent of other delivery organizations, other accrediting bodies have been developed to compete for the more specialized delivery mechanisms. Although some businesses have contracted directly with hospitals and other providers, the large business community has been more interested in looking at the plan level for evaluation of their insurers. This has allowed scrutiny of local sites for comparative and consistent performance in their multistate operations. Interest in the accreditation and measurement communities has increased recently with the slowdown of cost savings from discounting and negotiating fees. There clearly is recognition that the emphasis is now migrating very quickly to understanding the quality of the health care that purchasers buy.

The National Committee for Quality Assurance (NCQA) is an organization based in Washington, D.C., that is independent and nonprofit.[16] It reviews and accredits health maintenance organizations, as well as recently announcing an expansion of the reviews to other groups, such as preferred provider organizations (PPOs) and managed behavioral health organizations. The NCQA was founded in 1979 by the Group Health Association of America and the American Managed Care and Review Association, two Washington, D.C., trade associations that represent the managed care industry. It became independent of the trade associations in 1990 with the help of a grant from the Robert Wood Johnson Foundation. The NCQA's review process evaluates the following areas of a managed care system:

- quality assurance
- utilization management
- credentialing
- preventive health services
- members' rights and responsibilities
- medical records

With the demands from purchasers for data to support performance comparisons among plans, the NCQA, under the umbrella of its performance measurement group, developed the Health Plan Employer Data and Information Set (HEDIS). Though not a requirement for accreditation, many purchasing organizations use these data often in combination with some of their own requirements for purposes of comparisons among plans. Consumer demand for comparative information recently resulted in the public release of data for over 150 plans. Cary Sennett, NCQA's vice president for performance measurement, stated that HEDIS 3.0, the revised 1997 measurement set, will be an all-encompassing but efficient set of measures. "We are designing this set of measures to target not only commercial plans, but also those serving Medicare and Medicaid beneficiaries," Sennett stated, "and to pay much more attention to the issues of chronic and acute care."[17(p 2)] The previous HEDIS data set was criticized for insufficient development of outcome measures and for a primary emphasis on process measures used to measure outcomes by proxy.[18] The 1997 HEDIS 3.0 revision is intended to address this area of concern but appears in its final form to incorporate actual outcome data only to a modest degree. At present, there is no national database to collect data from plans, although there have been suggestions that this might be established. Consequently, most of the pooled data rests with the requesters, as well as with some consulting firms who have developed databases as a method for serving their customers.

The Joint Commission started accrediting managed care organizations in 1987 but stopped in mid-1990, in part because of insufficient demand. Subsequently, in 1995, it developed new standards for managed care networks and reentered the marketplace. As a part of the Agenda for Change that President Dennis O'Leary had initiated almost 10 years previously, the accreditation standards were functionally based and adaptable to a variety of managed care organizational entities. As an accreditor of over 16,000 organizations of various types, the Joint Commission places substantial emphasis on individual components of service delivery (like hospitals, long-term care delivery sites, and home health agencies). This contrasts with the NCQA approach, which requires managed care organizations to implement their own standards of participation for any components not accredited by a recognized organization. Although the largest number of plans have been accredited by NCQA, a growing number of organizations are selecting the Joint Commission. The major performance areas examined by the Joint Commission are

- patient rights and organizational ethics
- assessment of patients
- care of patients
- patient and family education
- continuum of care
- improving organizational performance
- leadership
- management of environment of care
- information management
- infection control
- governance
- organization management
- medical staff
- nursing[19]

In 1997, the Joint Commission announced its own performance measurement approach as the first performance measurement requirements actually placed on provider bodies. It labeled the approach as ORYX™ and defined the requirements for hospitals and its network program at this time. The system is in concert with the Joint Commission's direction of incorporating performance measures as a part of the continuous accreditation process. Accredited entities, by collecting and implementing performance measures, must demonstrate that they have used this information in actual changes in process and treatment. For the network program, the entities will not provide this information to a database, since none currently exists, but will be expected to demonstrate its use in their own networks. The networks may select from HEDIS measures for health plans, Joint Commission measures for acute care services, Foundation for Accountability measures for health plans, University of Wisconsin measures for long-term care services, or University of Colorado measures for home care services.

The Accreditation Association for Ambulatory Health Care (AAAHC) primarily affects such components of managed care as ambulatory centers, surgery centers, medical groups, and other entities that contract with health plans. The Utilization Review Accreditation Commission (URAC) has been in the business of accrediting utilization review organizations, many of which operate in conjunction with HMOs. They are entering the field of network accreditation and outlining standards for PPOs, HMOs, physician hospital organizations, independent practice associations (IPAs), and integrated delivery networks. This is not an exhaustive list by any means. However, it clearly indicates the growing interest for organizations to provide some level of consistency by meeting standards and measures established by external organizations that is being required by the payers of the services.

The most recent organization to emerge in the measurement contest is the Foundation for Accountability (FACCT). The driving force in the formation of FACCT was the Jackson Hole Group, led by Paul Ellwood, MD. This group included public and private purchasers representing over 80 million covered lives, as well as consumer representatives. It represented individuals fully committed to and active in the above organizations who, as purchasers, were frustrated by the fact that so many developed outcome measures were being incorporated too slowly by the accrediting bodies and by the fact that the data collected could not help them differentiate health improvement comparisons across plans. Contributions from the government and private corporations started the foundation, whose goal was to use the leveraging power of the purchasers for plans and measurement bodies to incorporate outcome measures for specific diseases and populations that the foundation would itself develop. According to David Lansky, FACCT president, the direction has been to stimulate the continuing reform of the health system by presenting these outcomes of performance to public scrutiny in terms that matter to consumers, patients, and purchasers.[20] The organization was established formally in 1996 and by the end of the year had produced three disease-specific sets— breast cancer, depression, and diabetes—and two populationwide topics, health risks and satisfaction. As described, the organization is focused on measurement and not accreditation. Incorporation of at least some of these measures has been accomplished in private purchasing contracts, in statements of intent by governmental agencies such as the Health Care Financing Administration, and by accrediting bodies such as the Joint Commission and the NCQA. Time will determine the value derived from the measure sets, but the influence of the payer and consumer has been prominent again.

Perhaps some question arises in readers' minds about the relationship of accrediting bodies and performance measures to chronic disease management. As has been pointed out, disease management rests on data collection and the use of this for continuing improvement. Accrediting bodies arise as a result of pressure from purchasing entities for meaningful information and measures. As Dennis O'Leary, president of the Joint Commission states frequently, "The human condition wishes not to be measured" (personal communication, 1997). Ultimately, the measures that are of interest to answer the question of the value of managed care rest in large part on their ability to improve outcomes in the management of chronic disease. It is important, then, to recognize that the leverage of the accrediting bodies on suppliers of health care is derived from the wise purchaser and consumer.

EXAMPLES OF DISEASE MANAGEMENT PROGRAMS IN THE PURCHASING COMMUNITY

Factors including type of business, number of employees, employees' age and sex distribution, employee turnover rate, geographic characteristics of the employer, union or nonunion workplace status, and company organization, philosophy, and resources influence the decisions about how purchasers incorporate disease management into their overall health strategies. Selecting the areas to explore that are pertinent to a particular market or employer involves searching the data for high-cost, high-frequency entities for the possibility of effective interventions. Selecting the population is another significant factor. As Figure 9–3 shows, a mere 11% of health plan enrollees submit three quarters of the charges.[21] Effective quality initiatives can be a successful driver for plans' reenrollment intentions of their members as well as general satisfaction. Effective disease management strategies manifest themselves as interest in patient welfare for plans in highly competitive cost-driven markets, as shown in Figures 9–4 and 9–5.

Selecting the disease entities to target for the largest impact rests on selecting data and viewing it in different ways. Heart disease always becomes a primary target when viewed relative to other disease processes. The financial impact as well as the mortality associated with heart disease is shown in Figures 9–6 and 9–7.

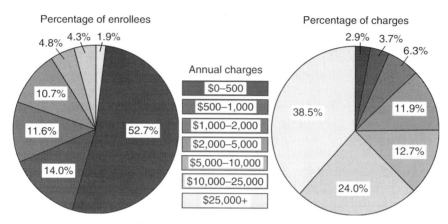

Figure 9–3 Picking the Targets for Outcomes Management. A mere 11% of enrollees submit three quarters of the charges. *Source:* Copyright Business & Health, made possible by a professional grant from Hoechst Marion Roussel.

The following demonstrates some of the approaches by different corporations and vendors currently reported in varying levels of detail. Although these are all reported as disease management programs, they contain variable elements of the concept as described.

An example of a thorough planning strategy is provided by the Sara Lee Corporation, which has developed a complete planning model to address the needs of its particular business units.[22(pp 7–12)] Its business units are widely distributed geographically and represent varying sizes and types of work. Obviously, one approach does not fit all. The benefit and health professionals, as a step in baseline measurements, attempt to collect data on health care claims, employee turnover rates, productivity measures, absenteeism rates, disability claims, and employee priorities. They created a table showing the selection of health improvement initiatives by demographics that delineates potential interventions for various population attributes (Table 9–1).

Of interest are the categories developed for initiatives. Disease management is a stand-alone category that identifies the targets as "large cases" for case management in all ages. Chronic case management applies only to a young population with low turnover. This demonstrates how purchasers, while understanding the need for long-term strategies, will focus, in many cases, on the more immediate returns that can justify a return on their investment. The table, of course, is a consolidation of the many factors reflected in their decisions about potential interventions.

Another example of a corporation that has created an initiative to control its health care costs while ensuring a high level of quality is the Hershey Foods com-

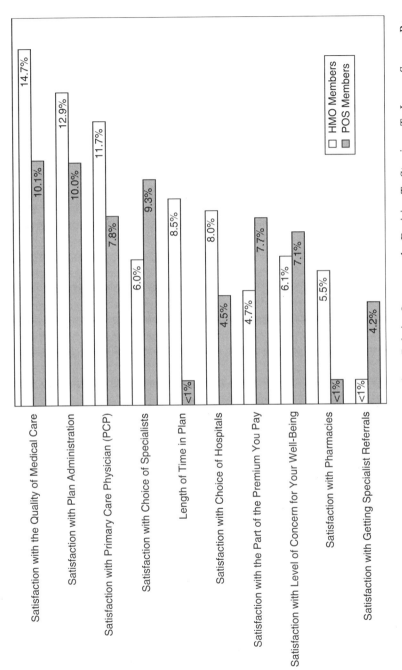

Figure 9–4 Key Factors That Affect Reenrollment Intentions: Relative Impact on the Decision To Stay in or To Leave. *Source:* Reprinted with permission from *1995 Ciba Geigy Reprt on Member Satisfaction Within Managed Care*, p. 16, © 1995, Venicom Custom Publishing.

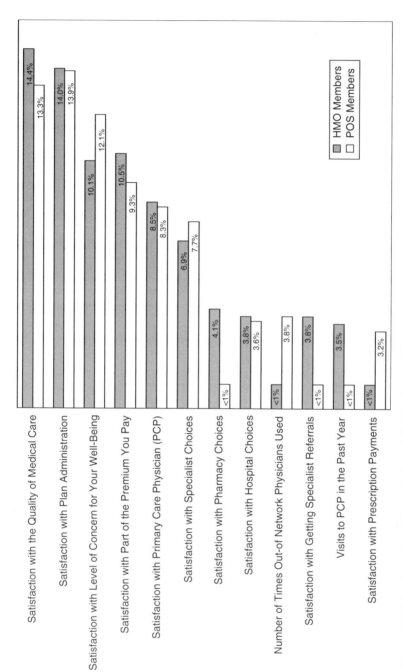

Figure 9–5 Most Important Drivers of Overall Satisfaction: Relative Impact on Overall Member Satisfaction. *Source:* Reprinted with permission from *1995 Ciba Geigy Report on Member Satisfaction Within Managed Care*, p. 22, © 1995, Venicom Custom Publishing.

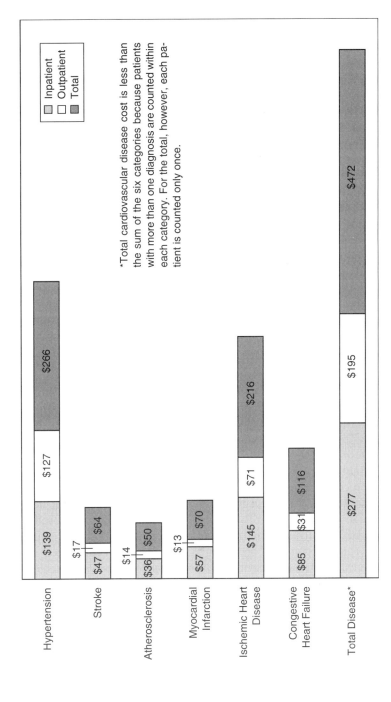

*Total cardiovascular disease cost is less than the sum of the six categories because patients with more than one diagnosis are counted within each category. For the total, however, each patient is counted only once.

Figure 9–6 Cost per Covered Life of Cardiovascular Conditions. *Source:* Copyright Business & Health, made possible by an educational grant from Bristol-Myer Squibb Company.

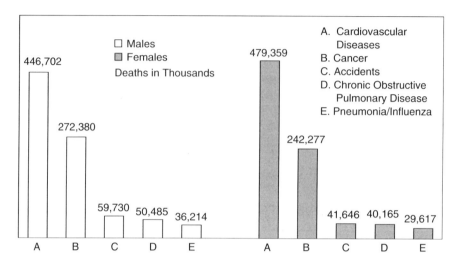

Figure 9–7 Leading Causes of Death, 1991. *Source:* Copyright Business & Health, made possible by an educational grant from Bristol-Myer Squibb Company.

pany in Hershey, Pennsylvania. Like John Deere, it has elected to build its own managed care network.[23] A dramatic increase in health care costs from 1989 to 1994 prompted it to consider different approaches to control. Its analysts used a data approach to identify selected providers with information gained from the Pennsylvania Health Care Cost Containment Council. By using a cooperative approach with various key players, including the union, the company has built a network and a process that allows for a partnership approach. Although the process has not always gone smoothly, Hershey has found effective mechanisms to manage information provided by the council to influence the management of procedures and processes in a solution-oriented way.

A broad variety of health interventions is included in the "discipline approach" of the Whitman Corporation.[22(pp 12–16)] These interventions required developing strong relationships between employees and primary care providers. Significant data collection and integration of these data by the company internally help select the interventions, which are mediated by the company's insurance carriers but are directed at the employee and the provider. The discipline approach includes financial incentives such as rewards dependent on compliance with a disease management regimen. In the company's arrangement with the provider for care counselors, there is a financial penalty for not engaging the health counselors during the decision-making process for an illness episode. A strong relationship is required with these counselors, who have the authority to initiate flexible benefits. The

Table 9–1 Health Improvement Initiatives: Selection by Demographics

Population Characteristics	Wellness Strategy	Demand Management Strategy	Disease Management Strategy
Older, longer service, low turnover	Focus on blood pressure, smoking, weight, exercise if justified by data	Analyze data for potential high utilization; focus on areas of high utilization	Analyze data for potential high utilization; focus on areas of high utilization
Older, high turnover	Minimal	Focus on access at time of illness to prevent problems from being overly expensive	Case management of large cases
Young, low turnover	Health education, prenatal care, preventive services	Focus on access at time of illness to prevent problems from being overly expensive	Case management of large cases and chronic diseases
Young, high turnover	Prenatal care	Seek out efficient health plans	Case management of large cases

Source: Reprinted with permission from *Encouraging Employee Involvement and Responsibility in Health Care,* p. 11, © 1996, Midwest Business Group on Health.

most noteworthy aspects of this program are the care model and strong financial incentives and disincentives.

Pitney Bowes elected to introduce a chronic disease management program developed internally and directed to employees only. It was designed and delivered by its own in-house health staffs and included on-site services as well as changes in the benefits plans to encourage employee self-management.[22(pp 23–27)] The company has used internal data sources to help define the population as well as to evaluate their results on an ongoing basis. The program is an asthma management program that was selected by a survey of employees. Management felt that "the work site offers easy access to these individuals, and the intervention program is a natural progression from worksite screening and wellness programs that are already in place at Pitney Bowes."[22(pp 27–30)] The program offers self-management and monitoring options. Pitney Bowes used its data resources to show that the asthma program resulted in significant improvement in quality of life and functionality as measured by the Asthma Quality of Life Questionnaire, job performance productivity, and number of emergency department visits. This program introduces significant educational monitoring and self-management techniques, but the primary pharmaceutical and medical management rests with the personal physician.

First Chicago Corporation[24] developed a program internally addressing depression in the workplace. The occupational medical department, led by the Employee Assistance Program (EAP) manager, developed a database that integrated information from three sources: short-term disability, medical claims, and EAP referral services. Department personnel elected to focus their activities on the workplace, which accounted for over half of all cases and allowed for ease of intervention. In addition to specific interventions, they made changes in their benefit design related to mental health benefits by allowing direct referral by their EAPs to mental health providers. They demonstrated their success by a reduction in the percentage of mental health costs that showed a drop of 5% from inception of the program in 1983 through 1995[22(p 26)] (see Figure 9–8). They are currently in the process of further quality measurements in the program. The significant aspect of this endeavor is the ability to incorporate disability data in the analysis that are unavailable in most health plans and that allow the possibility of defining productivity gains or losses. First Chicago is very interested in the productivity aspect of its program.

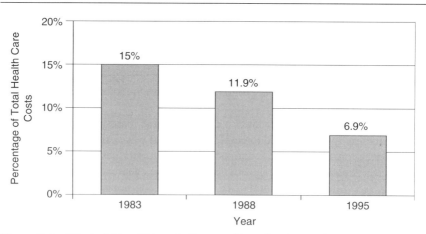

Figure 9–8   Effect of First Chicago's Program Targeting Depression on Percentage of Total Health Care Costs Constituted by Mental Health Care Costs. *Source:* Reprinted with permission from *Encouraging Employee Involvement and Responsibility in Health Care,* p. 26, © 1996, Midwest Business Group on Health.

Deere & Company[25] has been directly involved in health care delivery for over 15 years through its IPA-model HMO and staff-model HMO. The staff model contracting with the Mayo Clinic has introduced disease management for asthma and hypertension with plans for other disease-specific categories. "While primary care accounts for only a small part of the overall cost, primary care physicians, by their diagnostic referral, and intervention patterns, control about 80 percent of how money gets spent," says Robert Nesse, vice chairman of Mayo's family practice division. "So both Deere and BHCAG (Business Health Care Action Group in Minneapolis) have chosen to move upstream."[26 (p 69)] They have invested heavily in a clinical information system with an electronic medical record capability because they feel it is indispensable to disease management. While they acknowledge the ability to accomplish this in their staff-model group, they have identified a more daunting challenge in their larger IPA. The ability to integrate the medical record into the information process is key to adequate measurement of outcomes of clinical management at the episode-of-care level. Integrated delivery systems are in the best position to effect this, and Deere is clearly in a leading position in the large employer community to effect it.

Carlson Companies of Minneapolis[26] has embarked on disease management, partly through its membership in the Business Health Care Action Group. It has representatives on committees that design practice guidelines, as in the case of mammography, with its managed care organizations. Its approach has been primarily directed toward activities in the business coalition and in-house health promotion programs.

While many may argue that management of high-risk pregnancy should not be considered disease management, or, for that matter, a disease, there has been considerable program development in this area by managed care organizations and other private vendors. Programs are often presented by health plans as an added cost to the purchaser. Home Depot Corporation used the March of Dimes "Babies and You" materials and a high-risk case management component from Health Risk Management (HRM) in Minneapolis.[26] It claimed a decline of 77% in pregnancy cases in which costs exceed $75,000. The service includes physician-to-physician communication and regular nurse care manager contact.

FUTURE CHALLENGES AND OPPORTUNITIES

One of the major challenges in discussing future disease state management programs lies in establishing and holding to disease management's definition. As long as the term has so many different meanings to such a wide array of vested interests, it is fair to say that it will be touted in any one of numerous forms for a long time. However, if we subscribe to the definition used in this chapter, which includes defined populations, information management, and continuous evaluation, there seem to be significant opportunities for it to have a marked impact on the well-being of populations affected.

While larger corporations may have the vision to recognize that long-term savings are in their best interests, the very nature of American business, large or small, demands short-term results. The promise of managed care has been realized at some level to purchasers by reduction of costs through discounting and limiting access. The promise of disease management in its totality will in fact be slow in realizing maximum economic effects. While there may be some short-term savings, as described previously in this chapter, they do not reflect the whole picture. Our expectations are for broad programs to improve the health of the population, and we have described only singular program efforts with short-term evaluations. Payoffs may be enormous but a long time in coming.[2] The small employer with a young population and high turnover may not view this very positively.

Disease management is dependent on huge information systems and databases.[27] Much of this information is resident in health plans, but often only in administrative data. Early attempts to automate health care information centered on financial transactions (e.g., claims processing). Most of the systems currently in place were designed for these billing-related purposes. Few actually incorporated clinical information. Claims data alone, many feel, are inadequate for disease management purposes because they fail to identify such important factors as severity of illness or variations in treatment.[28] Patient records containing detailed diagnosis and treatment information remain largely paper based. Because of the enormous cost and logistics of using paper files for disease management purposes, there is significant interest in moving toward an electronic medical record. Many barriers exist to the development of this record, but substantial progress is being made.

Others do not agree with this notion. Several models have been developed to use insurance plan claims data, as well as Medicare's National Claims History File, to create episode-of-care data. Regardless of the validity of the methodology, it is clear that collecting information from all of the providers on one patient represents a large challenge and a costly one. If it is ever to be effective, it must be expanded to include patient records—a more significant challenge. Purchasers are generally not aware of this cost. If they are, most consider it a part of doing business. They may be willing to consider additional costs for disease management resulting ultimately in savings, but broadly they expect this to result in some short- and long-term well-defined estimates.

Larger employers and some business coalitions hold large amounts of data that can be of great value in targeting populations at risk, monitoring the effectiveness of interventions, and measuring productivity. Formalized interest in the latter is just beginning to appear. Productivity measures require the investment of resources to accomplish several tasks. Measurement of productivity in relationship to disability means merging that database with others to provide appropriate information. Introduction of health status measures that correlate with the type of work done also requires resource investment. Although there is a willingness to enter into this kind of effort, only time will tell if the associated expenses and complexities will be a barrier.

Epstein and Sherwood point out the distinction between effectiveness and efficacy as critical to disease management.[29] Efficacy studies require well-defined control groups and are done prior to effectiveness studies. However, effectiveness studies may be observational or protocol driven. Employers may not be willing to have an intervention withheld from their population and may be unwilling to conduct a clinical trial to prove efficacy before disseminating the program. With a concurrent comparison group and within a rapidly changing environment, aging and other factors may confound the "before" and "after" comparisons. Figure 9–9 shows the spectrum of disease concepts reviewed by the authors and the manner in which they relate to each other.[29(p 836)] Providers will need sophisticated training to ensure that they understand the complexity of interactions and make appropriate decisions regarding their value.

Fragmentation of services to employee populations can be a serious barrier to overall health improvement. Many employers have purchased separate pharmaceutical and behavioral health care carve-outs. They are continually being confronted with offers from other health service entities. Although they all promise and generally have produced cost savings to employers, they create challenges to providers. Issues influencing the quality of care delivered across organizations are not frequently discussed. Fargason et al provide a comprehensive view of the factors to be considered in introducing health services that are delivered by a process of care that spans several service organizations.[30] They use spina bifida as a chronic pediatric condition representative of potential chronic disease entities that lend themselves to disease management. To point out the complexity, they note that the services of general pediatricians, orthopedists, neurosurgeons, developmental specialists, physical and occupational therapists, school systems, home nursing and health agencies, and other agencies are routinely involved in the care of these patients. Communication and coordination barriers, differences in organization values and mandates, and personality conflicts all contribute their own characteristics that must be overcome to achieve a high-quality outcome for the individual patient. Some approaches that Fargason et al suggest to overcome these barriers include structural approaches using specialty centers and interorganizational teams or task forces.[30] Group process approaches are also described that include recognizing time constraints, agreeing on a common purpose, minimizing appeals to the overriding altruism of those involved, establishing a negotiation framework, and finally building on success. It would behoove any party embarking on a disease management process to review this article, which provides some

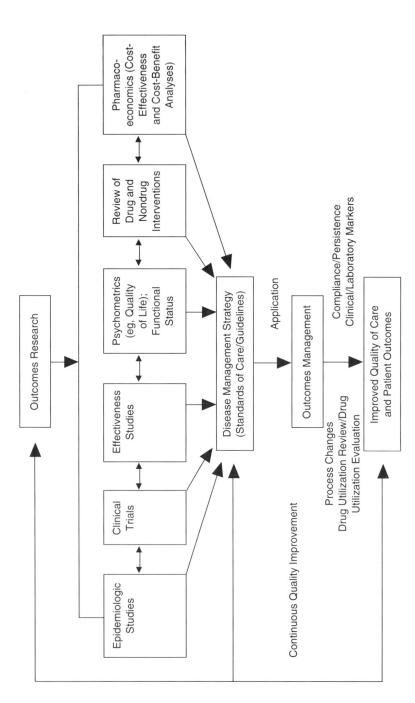

Figure 9–9 The Multidisciplinary Scientific Basis of Outcomes Research and the Manner in Which It Flows into Disease Management Programs. Continuous quality improvement of outcomes is the ultimate goal. *Source:* Reprinted with permission from Epstein and Sherwood, Outcomes Research to Disease Management: A Guide for the Perplexed, *Annals of Internal Medicine,* Vol. 124, pp. 832–837, © 1986, American College of Physicians.

insights into planning a program in a way that addresses these different barriers. From the patient's perspective, there may be difficulties in coordinating needed services. More purchasers are looking for ways to consolidate their internal management requirements by asking for such things as "24-hour coverage," i.e., purchasing health services from one vendor who must coordinate them. These 24-hour coverage plans include general health benefits, workers' compensation benefits, and disability benefits. Such programs will be very attractive to employers who are seeing their own internal management resources being pared by reengineering and reorganization efforts.

The opportunities for engagement in the process of disease management with significant contributions are there for the purchaser. Disease management embodies all of the elements of the total quality process. Benefits managers in the past purchased care on the basis of reimbursement methodologies based on information that required no accountability in health plans other than that based on actuarial models and level of benefits. Disease management requires an understanding of the typical disease drivers of cost and thus produces measures that can be more readily reported and understood. It allows for comparisons of management effectiveness of disease entities across health plans in lieu of proxy measures such as length of stay and number of visits. It broadens the possibility of measuring employee satisfaction not just with process issues, such as claim payments or telephone response time, but with satisfaction rates and with actual health data on chronic disease conditions, such as hospitalizations required, functional status of the individual, and quality-of-life outcomes. These become powerful tools to the purchaser in differentiating vendors.

Disease management requires enormous educational initiatives directed at patients, families, providers, caregivers, and employers. The incorporation of educational opportunities into occupational health programs can be an effective and positively viewed role for the purchaser. As new knowledge is gained from the disease management process, it must be communicated to the various stakeholders. The opportunities for incorporating this in health promotion, disability management, and often internal programs in the workplace can lead to a more holistic approach to employee well-being.

The jury on disease management is still out. There are many who say that there has yet to be a demonstrably positive report on the impact of these programs (but see Chapter 6 of this book). However, one must bear in mind, first, that the programs are too new to show any long-term effects, and second, that outcomes data of substance have yet to be reported in the peer review literature. The latter may have something to do with the reluctance of some groups to reveal proprietary data.

On the other hand, there continues to be full support in many quarters, based on nothing more than the belief that disease management is the core of what must be addressed to effect long-term health care improvement. Whatever the case, it would seem fair to view disease management as another transition in the evolving organization of health care in this country. Ultimately, "patient-centered care"—care that includes attention to primary through tertiary care in the preventive medicine model—would seem to be the most reasonable overall outcome (see Chapter 10). Patient-centered care interventions will address the working well, the acutely and chronically ill, and those with tertiary care needs. We now have the bits and pieces forming, and they need to be put together. The drivers in this endeavor will largely be the purchasing community.

References

1. Couch JB, Warshaw L. In: Couch JB, ed. *Health Care Quality Management for the 21st Century*. Tampa, Fla: American College of Physician Executives; 1991:387–397.
2. MacStravic S. Marketing or management: which way the future? *J Health Care Marketing*. 1996;16:10–13.
3. Kozma CM, Kaa KA, Reeder CE. A model for comprehensive disease state management. *J Outcomes Manage*. February 1997;4:4–8.
4. Medical utilization management. *DSM*. September 5, 1996;18:5–8.
5. Schear S. Detroit's new model for health care. *Bus Health*. February 1996;14:2–7.
6. Auto makers attack high health-care bills with a new approach. *Wall Street J*. December 9, 1996:A1,A6.
7. Couch JB. The total quality revolution. *Compensation and Benefits Manage*. 1992;8:44–48.
8. Sullivan S. Purchaser demands for quality and value. Presented at the meeting of the National Business Coalition on Health; September 1996; Orlando, Fla.
9. Wise D. Producing strength? The state of health care in America. *Business Health*. 1996;14: 39–42.
10. Sirio CA, Harper D. Designing the optimal health assessment system: the Cleveland Quality Choice (CHQC) example. *Am J Med Qual*. 1996;11:S66–S69.
11. Joint Commission on the Accreditation of Healthcare Organizations. Business Advisory Group Meeting; February 1997.
12. Pruett SH, Werner T, Hein J. The Cincinnati payer initiative. *Am J Med Qual*. 1996;11:S39–S41.
13. Disease management. *Healthcare Inf Cent*. December 1995;21:4–8.
14. Value Health, Johnson & Johnson collaborate to develop disease management products. *Health Care Strategic Manage*. 1995;18(8):9.
15. *Health Care Strategic Manage*. June 1995;13.
16. Woolsey C. Accreditation standards for HMOs winning praise. *Bus Insurance*. 1991:12.
17. NCQA's Committee on Performance Measurement: taking HEDIS to the next level. *Qual Matters*. Fall 1995:2.
18. Dimmitt BS. Managed care organizations are increasingly seeking a stamp of approval from an independent organization: does it matter which group does the job? Do employers care? Should they? *Bus Health*. 1995;13:38–43.

19. Joint Commission on the Accreditation of Healthcare Organizations.

20. Lansky D. Accountability update. *Accountability Action*. Foundation for Accountability 1996;1.

21. *Bus Health*. 1996;14(suppl 13):16.

22. Midwest Business Group on Health. *Encouraging Employee Involvement and Responsibility in Health Care*. Fairfax, Va: Severyn Healthcare & Publishing; 1996.

23. Tilley S, Bomberger D, Ackroyd T, Smith A, Hamory B. Data initiatives: building a managed care network utilizing clinical performance data. *Am J Med Qual*. 1996;11:S22–S26.

24. Terry K. Disease management: at these companies, the future is now. *Bus Health*. 1995;13:73–76.

25. Strategies for quality care and lower costs. *Bus Health*. 1995;13:28–32.

26. Disease management continuous quality improvement. *Bus Health*. 1995;13:65–76.

27. Bazzoli F, ed. Putting the Pieces Together. *Health Data Management*. 1 January 1996; 29–37.

28. Sylvestri MF. Health care informatics: the key to successful disease management. *Med Interface*. May 1996;94–99.

29. Epstein RS, Sherwood LM. From outcomes research to disease management: a guide for the perplexed. *Ann Intern Med*. 1996;124:832–837.

30. Fargason CA Jr, Ashworth CS, Haddock CC. Quality in the interorganizational setting. *Am J Med Qual*. 1995;10:3–9.

CHAPTER 10

Disease Management As Patient-Centered Care

David Levy

Throughout history, there have always been patients and healers. For the most part, healers and healing (in whatever form) have been central to the growth of civilizations and the evolution of cultures. In fact, helping the sick is so much a part of any given culture that the systematic organization of the delivery of healing is a mirror of the culture's core values.

This chapter will describe the return of our health care delivery system to patient-centered care. One must say "return," since its straying from that path over the last two decades has been anomalous to our culture and largely a result of economic and technologic forces that are just now coming back into balance. Disease management, a recently coined yet already ubiquitous term, is based on the tacit acceptance that all good health care is necessarily patient centered.

The essential values of the health care delivery system for those who use it are relief from pain and suffering, possible prevention or cure of illness, promotion of healthful longevity, and, above all (and not to be easily dismissed), doing no harm. It is remarkable that none of these values is rooted in technology or objectivity. Indeed, they are really a collective reflection of what any one of us feels we need at any moment. Many in our culture receive legitimate healing outside traditional medicine altogether, as in prayer and alternative medicine. The recent rise in the popularity of the latter despite tremendous advances in science and technology may be viewed as a measure of the inattention of traditional medicine to patient-focused values.

Healing and medicine are simply services available to the general population. Who chooses to avail him- or herself of these services, and under what conditions, relates to behavior that is driven by their perceived value measured against a variety of social and economic inputs. This chapter will review the history of health care management in the past few decades from a marketplace point of view, examine the results and conditions that have necessitated a new paradigm, and make the case that patient-centered care closes the loop and represents a return to basic values in the health care delivery system.

HISTORY OF HEALTH CARE MANAGEMENT

Marketplace Dynamics: Risk and Reward

In the early part of the century, receiving personal (as opposed to public) health care services came as a result of either a purchase with cash or barter or a charitable gift. There was no doubt concerning who was the focus of care or who judged its quality: the patient. There was also no doubt about who felt responsible for the patient's well-being: the treating physician. The patient asked for and received. The healer gave. Virtually no physician or hospital refused to give, and those who could afford to pay made up for those who could not. This medical tradition of charity is so deeply ingrained in the profession that even today it is considered unethical for hospitals to turn away the poor. Hospital privileges for physicians in large centers still almost always require the donation of some portion of time to charitable clinics.

Health insurers did not exist. No treatment was so expensive that it could not be had for a fee or charity. Most physicians would absorb the risk of nonpayment for services. Furthermore, all hospitals were funded through charity of one type or another, and maintenance of infrastructure was easily accomplished. It is safe to say that each physician and hospital operated as a little insurance company, bearing risk and striving to provide services directly to patients. Patients were the final arbiters of quality, making judgments with respect to value as treatment progressed.

The major advances in life expectancy were results of public health measures. Acute care technology was essentially supportive. Most patients died of infection or heart failure and died at home. Health care was not a right but a privilege.

At the center of the patient-physician relationship was trust, namely, the willingness of patients to accept that physicians always put their interests ahead of self-interest.[1] That combination of professional competence and a fiduciary ethic was extremely simple to adhere to in an era of low technology and personal responsibility for the financing of care. Patients chose treatment plans for medical conditions in the belief that to do otherwise was more risky. Physicians expanded their practices by offering professional services that engendered trust and objectivity and that met patients' and families' needs. The notion that health care could be anything but patient centered was absurd.

After World War II, the United States saw economic, social, and technological changes that dramatically altered the health care industry. Robust economic growth, the emergence of health insurance as an employee benefit, the social transformation of health care from a privilege to a right (symbolized by the ambitious Medicare program passed by Congress in 1965), and the rapid expansion of medical technology all contributed to what became medical hyperinflation in the 1970s. A massive industry (now close to 15% of the Gross Domestic Product) was created.

As a result of the hospital's becoming a greater focus of care in the 1930s and its increasing inability to bear its own risks, hospital insurance was born. Likewise, in the case of physicians, with the growing costs of medical education and the maintenance of a private practice, risk bearing for the cost of patients' care was possible only with a steady stream of paying patients. This problem was solved when employers (through private insurance) and the federal government (via Medicare and Medicaid) offered third-party payment for an increasing percentage of total benefits covered. Furthermore, the reimbursement rates to physicians were set at what was termed "usual and customary" fees, typically the 80th percentile of what physicians billed in the community. The result had patients almost completely insulated from health care costs and physicians with no fiduciary responsibility in the relationship. This led to medical inflation amounting to three times the consumer price index during the middle 1980s to early 1990s.

The fundamental nature of health insurance also changed. Insurance is usually thought of as a mechanism to protect from untimely and risky events such as catastrophic illnesses, motor vehicle accidents, or natural disasters. In lieu of a national health program similar to that of other industrialized countries, which broadened health insurance benefits to include coverage for routine, episodic, self-resolving, and preventive care, more and more benefits were provided by employers. They became small proxies for the entire health agenda of their working populations and their families. Insurance in the true sense disappeared, since the vast majority of premium costs was allocated to predictable and recurrent consumption. Health insurance, for the most part, had become a tax-preferred savings program provided by employers and the federal government to about three quarters of the U.S. population. But there was an ever-growing group of professionals clamoring to draw on those accounts, which by the mid-1990s had increased almost to $1 trillion annually. Getting everyone into the fund became a political issue that culminated in the failed federal health insurance reform initiative of 1993 and 1994.

Far more than could be included in this chapter could be said about the social and political consequences of the very existence of such a massive pool of money for the purposes of something as subjective as "health." Suffice it to say that the process that determined the right to draw on the money and the reasons for doing so became an industry in itself. Provider groups such as professional societies and hospitals, manufacturers such as pharmaceutical and device companies, and patient advocacy groups all jumped into the gold rush. Podiatrists lobbied for the same rights to cut as orthopedists (at least below the ankle). Psychiatrists had their exclusivity on mental health eroded by psychologists, who in turn had it diminished by social workers. Mental health advocacy groups succeeded in convincing legislators that most people, during the course of their lives, will suffer from mental illness that will require treatment. Patients with chronic back pain demanded hot tub reimbursement as an alternative to neurosurgery. Massage therapists asserted that they could treat cancer pain as well as oncologists. New technologies spawned new devices that in turn legitimized care by virtue of the right to draw on the fund. Ultrasound in pregnancy, cardiovascular stress testing, home monitoring of all types, and even Swan-Ganz cardiac catheterization are but a few examples. An entire durable medical equipment industry grew around the Medicare-allowable charges. The list goes on and on.

Though many have chronicled the evolution of our current health care industry from a wide variety of historical, economic, and technological perspectives, it is useful to examine the changes in what is surely the center and the locus of value of the health care system: the patient-physician relationship. Trust—the combination of professional competence and fiduciary responsibility providing the basis of the essential relationship between a physician and patient—became eroded by competing interests.

Professional competence used to be easy to judge. After World War II, it was judged by a medical degree from a licensed medical school and a general internship. Later, qualifications became residency completion, then board certification. Somewhere along the way, the granting of hospital privileges became an indicator. Attorneys got involved to the extent that a national database was established to track medical malpractice claims against individual physicians. Today, some even believe that the managed care plan should take responsibility for the assessment of competence.[2]

Professional competence has also become confused with technical competence. With the proliferation of medical technologies, excellence at doing something has supplanted the "if, why, and when" in the patient's best interest. Medical procedures became highly reimbursed, whereas cognitive skills did not.

The traditional fiduciary role of the physician dissolved as most care became prefunded, with little or no value testing required from the patient. Rather than being challenged every day concerning the value received for services, physicians were encouraged to produce services. Instead of thinking carefully about the consequences of services produced, patients just demanded them. Rising patient expectations generated more services, which in turn produced even greater demand. This undermined the traditional long-term nature of the patient-physician relationship and replaced it with a short-term, service-centered view. The most important question a doctor should have been asking—"How can I help solve your problem, without hurting you, so that you can live best?"—had been transformed to "What can I do for you now?" A patient without regard for the cost of services and a physician who is guaranteed payment for any number of services at any price constitute a recipe for a problem worse than inflation—the undermining and dissolution of the traditional values of our health care.

Marketplace Response: Price and Utilization Control

The natural marketplace response to the explosion of volume and price of services was volume and price controls. Driving this movement were large employers who, with the passage of the Employee Retirement Income Security Act of 1974 (ERISA), found it much less expensive to self-insure their employee and beneficiary pool, for whom every saved dollar went directly to the bottom line.

The first source of costs to be addressed was volume, specifically that of the most expensive site in the system, the hospital. The standard industry fare that evolved in the 1970s was hospital precertification, continued-stay review (CSR), discharge planning, and large case management. These volume controls, which became collectively known as utilization management, describe a set of activities carefully designed to assess the eligibility of services under a benefit plan, their appropriateness with respect to site of care, and their subsequent coordination to prevent excessive and unnecessary services. The effectiveness of traditional utilization management on service volume is controversial. There is no doubt that significant volume reductions did occur, especially in hospitals and communities with egregiously high hospital utilization rates. However, volume shifted to nonmonitored sites, such as outpatient medical and surgical suites, and overall volume of services increased. Medical inflation persisted.

The next attempt at volume reduction came from the development of rule-based expert computer systems designed to address the appropriateness of the care itself, rather than just the appropriateness of the site of care. These computer algorithms were procedure-focused (knee arthroscopy, magnetic resonance imaging [MRI] scanning, Caesarean section, cardiac catheterization, etc). They were produced with leading medical and surgical specialists as advisors. They enjoyed early market success in the late 1980s and early 1990s but waned in popularity as other, more cost-effective strategies gained importance.

Reducing price on units proved to be a slippery task. Fixing fees for a certain level of service led to widespread gaming of the system, as in "upcoding," or charging for a higher level of a similar service, and "unbundling," or billing separately for each task within a global service. Replacing hospital admissions with outpatient services was no problem. Soon outpatient surgical suites were priced higher than inpatient facilities. The introduction of the diagnosis-related group (DRG) method of payment to hospitals by the Medicare program in 1983 was a successful effort to pay hospitals on the basis of specific diagnoses rather than on units and price per unit. For the first time since the invention of health care insurance, hospitals were at risk again, and they learned to become more efficient within the prescribed diagnostic groupings.

In the late 1980s, with medical inflation still romping along in the double digits, an extremely significant set of events took place between the traditional payers (large self-insured employers) and their third-party administrators (the large insurance carriers). Rather than acting as pass-through claims payers returning medical inflation directly back to the carriers, employers demanded that that these third parties assume some of the risk of utilization and price controls through premium and medical cost guarantees. Usual and customary fees no longer applied, for all the carriers scurried to enlist physicians, hospitals, and other providers in their delivery networks. In return for accepting fixed monthly premiums based on panel size and discounted fees, physicians were offered to insured employees as "participating providers." The relative oversupply of physicians in urban and suburban areas was fertile territory for this kind of activity. For the first time, the professional taboo of price competition among physicians had been overcome.

A significant impediment to moving employees into more "managed" care plans was the fact that most Americans demanded the right to choose their own physicians in times of need. Many patients felt that networked provider plans were adequate for routine care but that the better-established, highly specialized, and often university-based physicians needed for specialized care were not available. This problem was solved by the invention of an extraordinary insurance product called the point-of-service plan, or POS. Originally conceived as a transitory step toward tightly managed networks, this product was named for the ability of the beneficiary to receive different benefits depending on the point in the delivery system where he or she accessed the care. Thus, the worried well and those who needed routine care could use participating providers with extremely low access fees and, when terribly sick, had the choice to leave the network, though with higher attendant costs. The peace of mind this gave to the vast majority of the healthy population, together with low-cost access to routine care, opened the way for this new kind of managed care or, more aptly, new kind of benefit plan. In the last 5 years, the majority of the commercially insured population joined a managed care organization with a POS plan or "open-model" plan. Closed-panel or staff-model HMOs experienced little growth during that time. This very large movement of premiums into managed-care plans further strengthened carriers' ability to put pressure on provider fees and hammer away at supply-side costs.

Price and utilization controls, however, had their limits. They have never been successful in the control of inflation in other parts of a free economy, and there is no reason to suspect that they could have enduring value in the health care system. The only way to control cost and utilization is to somehow reinject fiduciary and consumptive responsibility into the patient-physician relationship, as in a more normal marketplace. This would ensure the responsible use of volume by providers at competitive prices, with demand appropriately mediated by patients sensitive to the value received.

In recent years, with heightening competition among managed-care organizations, this has begun to happen. Managed care companies have forced fiduciary responsibility back onto providers by transferring large segments of the premium risk to them. Hospitals have accepted global per diem rates adjusted by site of care in the hospital, case rates, and even capitated rates (ie, fixed monthly fees on a defined population to cover all health care costs). Physicians have also responded in kind by accepting larger and larger slices of risk. What began as accepting risk for only those services they could provide has grown to premium risk accepted for services provided by others, such as hospitals, ancillary care, chronic care, and drug benefits. When services are combined in this way, the arrangement is referred to as *global risk* or *global capitation*. A whole new industry has developed in the past 3 years: physician practice management companies, or PPMs, whose basic mission is to help physicians manage global capitation. Once again, the medical community has begun to bear fiduciary responsibility for health care services.

How does all of this relate to the patient-centeredness of care and the strength of the patient-physician relationship? As described, the dissolution of trust began with relief of both patients and physicians from their fiduciary responsibilities in the purchasing and delivery of care. Decisions made by patients concerning value, as based on their own needs, were supplanted by decisions made by external arbiters acting on behalf of payers to limit the right to draw on prefunded premium for every patient. As a result, physicians were no longer doctors, but providers. Disease management is all about refocusing the health care system on patients with medical problems, doing the very best for patients in the moment and over time, and showing economic value and enhanced well-being as a result.

The New Medical Marketplace: Providers at Risk

It is impossible to overemphasize the significance of the return of risk to providers as a key event in the evolving medical marketplace. This is not without serious ethical concerns, the most obvious being the incentive to produce fewer-than-necessary services. However, even more significantly, this event has decisively moved the economic focus away from the site of care and placed it squarely on the patient, irrespective of where he or she may be in the system. Once again, the physician is closely invested in his or her patients' well-being in a deeper way. The expectations of value for services have a much further horizon than the office visit, hospital stay, or outpatient procedure.

In the new paradigm, health care financing has become a flow of premium downstream to providers. Health care benefit plans are being rewritten to describe relationships in the context of physicians and patients rather than payers and beneficiaries. Utilization management in the traditional sense is an anachronism. Finally, old and insufficient measures of performance on cost, quality, and patient satisfaction need redefinition.

Thomas S. Kuhn, in *The Structure of Scientific Revolutions,* clearly describes the role of crisis (such as uncontrollable health care costs) in initiating paradigm shifts. He describes well the normal course of events: old solutions are insufficient and new ones are sought. New views have both destructive and constructive elements; old rules are discarded and replaced with new ones. The emergence of new theories generally is preceded by a period of pronounced professional insecurity.

The next section will describe the insufficiencies in the old delivery system from the perspectives of patients, physicians, and payers. The last section will describe the new paradigm and how stakeholders will need to adapt to it.

INSUFFICIENCIES OF THE OLD VIEW

Imagine a sick patient with terminal cancer who spent 2 years seeking and receiving the best treatments that medical science has to offer. More treatment was proving to be less curative and painful, and he was considering stopping treatment in order to experience a better quality of life in his remaining time. The patient had long given up his relationship with his primary care physician who had discovered the initial lesion in favor of his attending oncologist and surgeon, who were dealing with the problem definitively.

The previous 2 years had gone pretty smoothly, once the system was well understood. The patient was properly referred to a surgeon who participated in his employer's health benefits network. Despite some negotiating on the surgeon's part with the benefit plan representative on the need for the procedure to be conducted inside or out of the hospital, the procedure was done as a "23-hour" case, thus avoiding a "real" hospital admission. The surgeon also had to agree to the benefit plan's fee structure. A tissue diagnosis was made, and the patient was referred to an oncologist.

The oncologist also participated in the health care network, but before receiving any care beyond an office visit, she had to consult with a nurse representing the employer's benefit plan to get agreement on the appropriateness and site of care. The oncologist was a published author and investigator in the area of the patient's histopathology, and the utilization management nurse had been in administrative medicine for over 15 years.

The patient, grateful to have one of the leading oncologists taking care of him, immediately accepted the standard chemotherapeutic and radiation protocol offered. The oncologist told him that current treatment protocols, given many times in her office, were promising. There was a significant chance for tumor regression, which the patient interpreted as a cure. Just before each treatment, the patient was sure to call the utilization management nurse for approval.

The patient did quite well initially, returned to work, and was as productive as possible. Unfortunately, after the fourth course of chemotherapy, the tumor started to grow again, and the oncologist recommended a different approach, using a mixture of several new agents. The new treatment had to be delayed a few weeks because it was not familiar to the utilization nurse. She had to review it with her boss, the medical director, who in turn needed to have several consultations with the treating oncologist. Although this was a little frustrating to the patient, he was reassured because so many people seemed to be concerned about his welfare.

This new treatment plan was much more toxic than the patient thought it would be. He could not return to work and felt extremely weak. The utilization management nurse arranged for a home health agency to help him right after his chemotherapy, but life was not progressing well at all. It was at about that time, despite hopeful signs from the oncologist, that he decided to have a long discussion with his wife about death and dying.

The patient and his wife had a long conversation about their hopes for the future, and he made it very clear from that moment that he was not interested in heroics. He would do his best to get better, given reasonable chances on therapies, but did not want to end his life in a hospital. The couple agreed that the next step was to have a conference with the oncologist to discuss whether to continue treatment, try another treatment, or stop completely.

The oncologist was not available until their next appointment in 2 weeks, since she was in Europe presenting a scientific paper. The covering oncologist had never met the patient and his wife and, because they had no real relationship, felt it would be best to wait for her. Their primary physician had not seen them for over a year and was not really up to speed on the disease or the treatment plan.

A week later, in the middle of the night, the patient woke up with shaking chills. His wife took his temperature, which was 104°F degrees orally, and rushed him to the hospital. The emergency room physician discussed the case with the covering oncologist, who ordered a septic workup and immediate admission. While in X-ray, the patient began to feel short of breath, and an arterial blood gas showed hypoxia. The chest X-ray indicated massive pneumonia. Blood gases worsened, and before dawn the oncologist asked for a consultation with a specialist in pulmonology. She strongly suspected adult acute respiratory distress, transferred the patient to the intensive care unit, intubated him, and corrected his blood gases. The next day, the utilization management nurse strongly agreed with the need and site of services. The patient did not do well. Despite intensive hemodynamic, antibiotic, and respiratory support, he expired after 5 days in the intensive care unit.

Everyone did his or her job. The physicians identified and treated the cancer with the best that medical science had to offer. The benefits representative audited the treatment plan, and the providers were paid. Hospital admissions and supposedly excess costs were reduced. Reports could be produced to document satisfactorily these activities.

This is not an unusual story. In fact, stories like this are representative of patients who account for at least one third of the total cost of the health care system. What they exemplify is a health care delivery system focused on treatments and treatment sites, not on the needs of a sick human being. The patient should be important. The illness is tangential.

Let us reexamine all aspects of this patient's journey with his illness to test the assertion that his medical management did not necessarily represent his best interests or those of the treating physicians or the health care benefit plan that paid for the care. Upon detection, the patient had a diagnostic excision of his lesion. Because a 23-hour admission was negotiated, a "real" admission was avoided, reducing the payer's admission and bed-day rates. However, there is at least an equal chance that this outpatient procedure cost more than its equivalent inpatient stay, particularly in light of acute care hospitals' cost shifting to less controlled outpatient environments. It is hard to say whether this patient would have been more comfortable not being shuffled in and out so quickly or whether he would have preferred to be at home.

Once the diagnosis was made, the patient was offered a treatment plan proffered by a leading specialist. Alternatives were not explored, and the patient accepted the plan "as is." He also gave up his relationship with his primary care physician. Most probably, no extensive discussion occurred regarding the patient's long-term view of his illness. The patient's participation in the decision making was minimal. The literature supports this notion: the further away from graduation, the less likely the physician is to support patient decision making.[3] Patients with shorter physician relationships participate less in decision making.[4,5]

As the treatment moved along, there were several conversations between the utilization management nurse and both the patient and the oncologist. The nurse had never met the patient or his family. When the tumor recurred and a new regimen was suggested, the utilization management nurse referred the case to the medical director. The discussion around the new plan with the medical director and the oncologist related to coverage and medical appropriateness. The focus was the care plan and the benefit plan, not the care plan and the patient with an illness. Physicians who are satisfied with their professional autonomy are more comfortable with patient-led decision making.[5] Here, physician autonomy was obviously constrained.

With the deterioration of his condition and the reduction of the quality of his life, the patient wanted to reevaluate his situation. He made his wishes clear to his wife, but the only physician with whom he had a relationship was not available for guidance or support. It is no surprise that when he became septic in a downward-spiraling clinical course, he landed in an intensive setting, where he expired[6] (see also Franklin Health–Oxford Health Plan, Patient-Centered Care Pilot, unpublished data, 1996).

One could not argue that for this patient, the outcome (not "only" death but the course of events culminating in the site of death) was less than optimal. What is not obvious is that the cost of care was greater than it should have been. Had the final episode of illness been properly managed, with the patient making choices with the support of the clinical team, the total illness would have cost the benefit plan less than it did. That final episode may have represented anywhere from 5% to 25% of the entire cost of the illness (Franklin Health–Ingersoll-Rand, internal data, 1993–1995).

The insufficiencies of the current paradigm as described above can be reviewed from the perspectives of the patient, physicians, and payer. The patient never had any real informed choice upon which he could base a treatment plan suitable to himself, and thus was not a part of the decision-making team. He had many interactions with a utilization management nurse, none of which changed the course of the treatment and illness. Worse, these represented lost opportunities to help the patient with his needs. Trying to change the course of treatment late in the illness required support and execution from his providers of care, but the requisite time, and perhaps interest, of his physician was not available. Finally, the terminal care events, once launched, were irrevocable.

The primary care physician was taken out of the equation early. Little or no feedback was forthcoming from the oncologist on the course of treatment. Home care was not coordinated through the primary care physician's office. It is difficult to assess whether this was a matter of lack of interest or lack of confidence on the part of the primary care physician. The oncologist was distracted on several occasions with interactions from the utilization management nurse and medical director of the benefit plan that involved negotiating for the site of care, with no tangible effect on the patient. Perhaps the oncologist's time would have been better spent with the patient and his wife. The oncologist, as a member of the benefit plan network, certainly had her fee discounted, but not by nearly as much as the extra cost generated by treatment the patient did not want. All the specialists during the terminal event did their jobs. All organ and physiologic systems were treated correctly and, as the utilization management company verified, at the right site.

The payer was generally blind to the actual course of treatments paid for by its benefit plans. Others were retained to determine eligibility, ensure coverage for specific services at specific sites, and pay claims. The payer received data on cost by provider type and service site utilization. In the managed care world, "report cards" on a variety of measures almost never address the conduct and content of care.

PATIENT-CENTERED CARE AS THE NEW PARADIGM OF HEALTH CARE MANAGEMENT

The clinical scenario described above should become less and less frequent in the foreseeable future. Once again, physicians are invested in their relationships with patients. Patients are also paying more attention, largely as a result of the rise of information technology and consumerism, making available for the first time highly complex and esoteric medical knowledge around which they can initiate and maintain their own decision making as well as make comparative judgments. In the future, they will pay even more attention as they share more in the real cost of care. In this new patient-centered world, different things will matter to patients, physicians, and payers. Definitions of value come full circle, back to the relief from pain and suffering, possible prevention or cure of illness, promotion of healthful longevity, and doing no harm.

Patients in this new paradigm will demand efficiency and quality, not office visits and prescriptions. Solving problems in the quickest and least expensive manner with the best results will drive physician and patient behavior. Choice will count more and more, particularly as well-informed patients demand the very best. The patient requiring open-heart surgery will know which hospital has the best results and insist on going there. The AIDS patient will demand the latest combination of antiviral agents, and, through a local support group, will push the envelope on what is best. The breast cancer patient will want to understand the five treatment choices available (three conventional and two experimental). The prostate cancer patient will not blindly have a prostatectomy. Pain control, activities of daily life, advance directives, and terminal care plans will all count for something. "Toll booths" (i.e., utilization management checkpoints, medications requiring a physician's prescription that can be bought over the counter, and laboratory tests by physicians and hospitals that may be performed as accurately and more quickly and cheaply by patients) will be avoided.

Table 10–1 shows the effect of patient-centered management on terminally ill patients enrolled in a large and prestigious managed care organization. Attending to needs at the service site (advance directives and health care proxies) was insufficient to drive treatment plan changes. Most important was the timing of patient-centered management: all of those well into their treatment plans who were referred late into the patient-centered program expired in the hospital[6] (see also Franklin Health–Oxford Health Plan, Patient-Centered Care Pilot, unpublished data, 1996). The majority of those patients referred to the program at an appropriate time in the course of their illness expired at an alternate site. The Patient-

Table 10–1 Patient-Centered versus Service Site Management in Terminal Illness

	Referral to Patient-Centered Program	
Quality Measure	*Timely*	*Late*
Advance directives	52%	60%
Health care proxy	59%	73%
Directives success:		
All directives followed	66%	67%
Most directives followed	5%	7%
Some directives followed	7%	6%
No directives followed	21%	20%
Place of death:		
Hospital (ICU or CCU)	9%	20%
Hospital	34%	80%
Inpatient hospice	11%	0%
Skilled nursing facility	5%	0%
Home	41%	0%

Timely intervention = 56 cases
Late intervention = 15 cases

Courtesy of Oxford Health Plans, Norwalk, Connecticut, and Franklin Health, Inc., Upper Saddle River, New Jersey.

Centered Care Pilot showed that two thirds of all severely ill patients in the program, when surveyed by an independent group, reported an enhanced quality of life as a result of patient-centered management.

Providers of care will now participate in the risk for the cost of an illness. In the hope of retaining patients, they will strive for highly satisfactory results. They will have stronger incentives to perform at higher quality and greater efficiency. The number of long-term relationships with patients will replace the number of services as a proxy for success.

The asthmatic who lands in the emergency room five times a month needs a more comprehensive approach by the physician or hospital at risk. Rather than ensuring that the emergency room is the best place for an adolescent with status asthmaticus, providers will pay serious attention to early risk identification and avoidance as a matter of economics as well as good medicine. The same is true for diabetics, whose prevention of renal failure with the use of angiotensin-converting enzyme (ACE) inhibitors is now of material importance to the physician group at risk. Perhaps aggressive behavior intervention and modification models (proven to be as or more effective at times than invasive strategies) will be offered to heart patients before angioplasty or bypass surgery.

Provider-driven creative solutions will emerge around internal cost management and getting patients the best care quickly. New data inputs will enable physicians to identify earlier and manage more closely clinical problems that may have otherwise been more complex. Polypharmacy in patients will be avoided, if at all possible. Unnecessary laboratory tests will not be ordered. Alternative treatments that have been shunned by the medical community but that may be effective in some patients, such as acupuncture, massage therapy, and chiropractic, may be used more.

A patient-centered cardiology program, aimed at those patients requiring invasive cardiology procedures shows how better choices for patients, based on objective data, can drastically improve the quality of care, yet reduce its cost. Figures 10–1 and 10–2 illustrate the migration from low-quality to high-quality cardiac centers for the beneficiaries of a large industrial concern after the inception of a patient-centered program (Franklin Health–GTE, internal data, 1992–1994). The majority of centers were paid on total-episode fees. Therefore, length of stay ceased to be a reimbursement issue and became one of a number of other quality measures.

Finally, the fundamentals of the delivery system will revert to health care's long tradition. The physician-patient relationship will again become central to health care. Physicians will understand that they provide the true value in the delivery system. With patient-focused management systems, they will be able to articulate very clearly how value is produced.

Payers, whether they are employers, government, or insurance companies, will surrender their need to intervene directly between their beneficiaries and

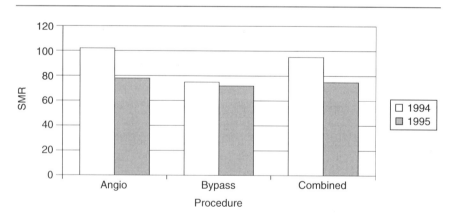

Figure 10–1 Standard Mortality Rate, 1994 versus 1995, after Cardiac Program Installed. Courtesy of Ingersoll-Rand, Woodcliff Lake, New Jersey, and Franklin Health, Inc., Upper Saddle River, New Jersey.

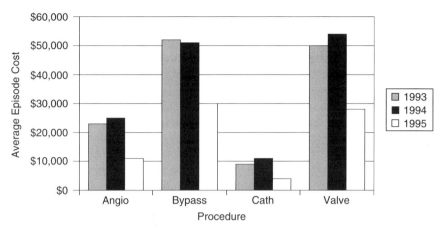

Figure 10–2 Average Episode Cost for Unmanaged Episodes (1993–1994) versus Managed Episodes (1995). Courtesy of Ingersoll-Rand, Woodcliff Lake, New Jersey, and Franklin Health, Inc., Upper Saddle River, New Jersey.

caregivers. Rather, their role will be to promulgate common and accepted measures of efficiency, quality, and effectiveness.

The new measures will only faintly resemble the old. Service site utilization rates (hospital days per 1000, admission rates per 1000, office visits per beneficiary per year, etc) will be replaced with measures that relate to patients: their illnesses, health outcomes, and satisfaction and the costs to them and their families.

Figure 10–3 and Table 10–2 show the cost reduction of patient-centered care management on several stage-adjusted diagnostic areas. Average severity-adjusted cost was reduced incremental to utilization management in the targeted diagnostic areas by over 11% when those very ill patients that would benefit from patient-centered management were chosen. From the same data, Figure 10–4 shows that cost was reduced an average of 29% for those cases managed directly.

Total plan costs will no longer be analyzed solely on an actuarial basis. Risk will be quantified on the prevalence of disease, severity adjusted within populations[7] (see also Franklin Health–Analytic System, unpublished data, 1996). Severity-adjusted disease measures will become the benchmarks. Comparative cost data will be available on physicians and hospitals that treat stage 3 breast cancer, or NYHA class 2 heart disease. Far less important than the cost and utilization of the site of care will be who can get the job done with the highest quality, satisfaction, and efficiency levels for a patient with a severity-adjusted level of disease. Pricing of health care benefit plans will move from an actuarial to epidemiologic plane.

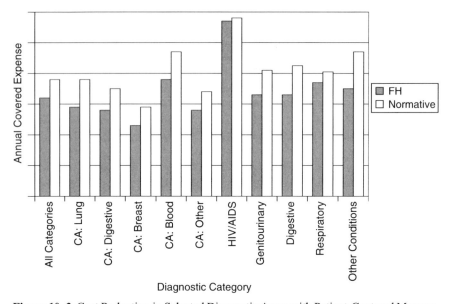

Figure 10–3 Cost Reduction in Selected Diagnostic Areas with Patient-Centered Management. Courtesy of HCIA, Inc., Baltimore, Maryland, and Franklin Health, Inc., Upper Saddle River, New Jersey.

Table 10–2 Cost Reduction in Selected Diagnostic Areas with Patient-Centered Management

MDG	FH Claimant Count	Adjusted Expenses Based on Comparison Data (in $)	Adjusted Savings (in $)	Adjusted Savings Percentage
Cancer: blood	107	8,228,744	(875,490)	−11.9%
Cancer: breast	117	6,919,269	(692,947)	−11.1%
Cancer: digestive	206	13,474,986	(1,385,620)	−11.5%
Cancer: lung	131	9,017,470	(1,272,051)	−16.4%
Cancer: other	375	23,997,853	(2,224,423)	−10.2%
Digestive	84	6,022,491	(781,203)	−14.9%
Genitourinary	105	7,494,689	(906,733)	−13.8%
HIV/AIDS	24	2,128,578	(34,074)	−1.6%
Other conditions	68	5,277,458	(853,271)	−19.3%
Respiratory	96	6,778,767	(304,047)	−4.7%
Grand Total	1313	89,340,305	(9,329,859)	−11.7%

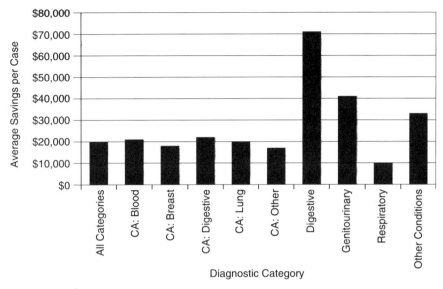

Figure 10–4 Average Savings per Case in a Patient-Centered Management Program. Courtesy of HCIA, Inc., Baltimore, Maryland, and Franklin Health, Inc., Upper Saddle River, New Jersey.

As a result of these new measures, management action will be less focused on population pool risk splitting, benefit plan "tuning," and cost-shifting. Attention will be focused more on identifying the medically manageable cost drivers inside a health care benefit plan and making sure they get managed against reliable and reproducible reporting. Figure 10–5 describes to a payer the net results of a patient-centered management approach on total plan costs (Franklin Health–Analytic System, unpublished data, 1996).

Outcome and quality today are mostly substitutes for efficacy—did it work, and how well? In the future, efficacy will be only one aspect of quality. Choice, pain, activities of daily living, and many more patient-centered measures, some subjective, will become important.

PUTTING IT ALL TOGETHER

As the paradigm shifts to traditional values in which the healer and his patient are at the center of the delivery system, it is useful to examine the roles of some of the players in the system today and in the future.

Figure 10–6 separates patients into three general claimant categories: the 90% who generate average annual costs less than $1200, the 9% who generate average costs greater than $6600, and the 1% or fewer with average annual claim costs in

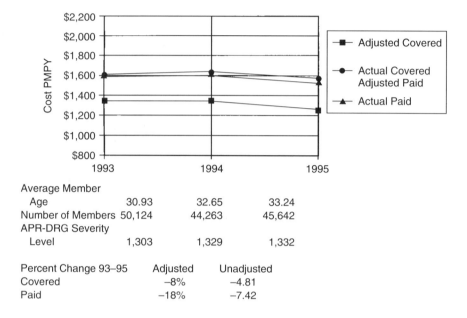

Average Member			
Age	30.93	32.65	33.24
Number of Members	50,124	44,263	45,642
APR-DRG Severity			
Level	1,303	1,329	1,332

Percent Change 93–95	Adjusted	Unadjusted
Covered	–8%	–4.81
Paid	–18%	–7.42

Figure 10–5 Severity-Adjusted Cost Trend, 1993–1995. Actual data, 50,000-member employer. Courtesy of Franklin Health, Inc., Upper Saddle River, New Jersey.

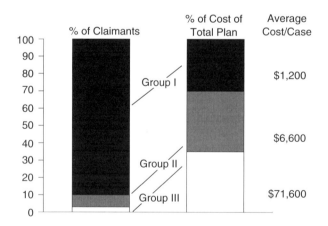

Figure 10–6 Claimant Types with Representative Claims Cost. *Source:* Franklin Health, internal data. Courtesy of Franklin Health, Inc., Upper Saddle River, New Jersey.

excess of $70,000. As can be seen, each group represents about a third of the total cost of care in the system.

Group I: The 90%

These patients are generally those with acute resolvable illnesses that are non-hospital or -facility based. They generally have small accidents, mild infectious diseases, and extremely low-grade chronic illnesses like migraine or low back pain. The worried well with nonspecified diagnoses and preventive well care are also included, as are the many patients with illnesses that resolve spontaneously without the need for medical intervention. These patients are the daily fare for busy primary care practitioners, including nurse practitioners and physicians' assistants.

In the old paradigm, the preferred management strategy was laissez-faire. Traditional utilization management was not worth the effort, since each episode of care was of fairly low cost and, measured against the value of external intervention, was not considered worthwhile. However, with a traditional fee-for-service system and little fiduciary responsibility, physician office visits could be excessive, while evading the usual scrutiny. For example, it was not uncommon for pediatricians to separate combined vaccines into individual visits. Multiple rechecks were requested for self-resolving illnesses.

Pharmaceutical manufacturers viewed the physician as the customer as opposed to the patient and hence took "medical education" into their own hands. Through off-site seminars (tax-deductible and sometimes free vacations), helpful minor office gadgets (ie, product promotion), and hospital-based continuing medical education credits (including expensive courtesy dinners), physicians were encouraged to prescribe a particular brand of anti-infective, antidiarrheal, anti–gastric acid, antihistamine, or muscle relaxant. The result was enormous abuse of these agents, many of which were not indicated or simply did not work for the prescribed conditions.

In the new world of medicine, fiduciary responsibility has been reintroduced. Physicians are paid fixed fees, not fees based on volume of services or on price. However, low access fees, the major additional benefit offered by POS plans, created enormous demand. The worried well and those with self-resolving ailments now have little or no financial barrier to a physician. Reducing office visits for these patients when possible is now of economic interest, provided that patients do not go directly to a higher-cost point of access, like an emergency department. Recognizing this as a business opportunity, the new industry of "demand management" has leapt into the health care scene. For a fixed monthly premium, a medical answering service staffed with nurses offers help on simple issues and steers patients away from emergency departments to physicians' offices or keeps them at home.

Reducing the cost of prescription drugs is now important for capitated physicians and capitated pharmacy benefit management companies (PBMs), which have carved out or assumed the risk of paying for all medications from the primary risk bearer, usually the managed care organization. The new notion of rational use of these medications has become important. The data that payers now see, such as the rank order of drug utilization by class of drug, prescribers, patients, and so forth, force important medical questions. For example, histamine-2 blockers for the treatment of gastric hyperacidity have traditionally topped the drug utilization list, yet much of that utilization has been completely unnecessary. Payers are now asking the PBMs to take the financial risk for this overprescribing, and PBMs are in turn creating demand reduction programs for these prescription drugs. Now the pharmaceutical companies, in the face of dramatic volume reduction, have successfully received FDA approval to sell these and other high-volume prescription items, such as nonsteroidal anti-inflammatory agents and antihistamines, over the counter without the need for a physician's prescription. These drugs are now advertised directly to the public, with payer indifference, since nonprescription drugs fall outside of health care insurance.

Group II: The 9%

This group of patients, with annual average claims costs of less than $7000, has more significant illnesses than those just described. These are patients who have well-controlled chronic diseases like asthma, diabetes, hypertension, hypercholesterolemia, colitis, multiple sclerosis, and connective tissue disorders. They may include those who need procedures such as childbirth, elective surgery for minor conditions like athletic injury, and cardiac catheterization. They may also have early-stage or low-grade neoplasm or HIV infection or may be in remission.

It is around this group of patients that the most intrusive external volume reduction has taken place. Hospital utilization rates used to be very high for this group, with admissions for workups and "tests" abounding. Much of this care has been moved to outpatient settings, yet these people still get an enormous amount of attention. These are the patients who have multiple and repeated imaging—fluoroscopy, chest X-rays, CAT scans, MRI scans, ultrasonography, nuclear medicine studies. They also have procedures—endoscopies, arthroscopies, pulmonary function testing. They get operated on early and often and have hysterectomies, tonsillectomies, cholycystectomies, polypectomies, and mastectomies. These are also patients who have neoplasms detected early and treated, or who, if the neoplasm is in remission, have biopsies and/or chemotherapy.

The variation of care that these patients receive around the country has drawn much attention.[8] Their overutilization of physician-driven services of questionable value was the early focus of traditional hospital and outpatient precertification. Early attention was given to the site of care, which was easily moved and priced in a compensatory fashion. Later, disease protocols and computer algorithms were developed with leading medical experts and then transformed to computer algorithms aimed to get physicians to behave similarly.

Office-based diagnostics flourished: fiber optics for peering into orifices, electronics for office-based ultrasound, echocardiography, cardiac monitoring, blood testing. Manufacturers, together with procedure-driven physicians, prospered. Even relatively difficult surgery like cholycystectomy was reinvented with the use of fiber optics as an outpatient procedure. The mark of a successful physician-businessman was one who could identify the number of patients with a particular medical problem seen in a prescribed period of time, quantify the number of new diagnostic tests designed for that problem that could be performed in his office, multiply the insurance-allowable reimbursement per procedure, and estimate in how many days, weeks, or months the investment on the new technology would be repaid and become profitable.

An interesting aspect of this patient group is how many are not optimally treated for common diseases that, if well treated, could mitigate or completely avoid downstream complications. Coronary artery disease is exemplary. The effect of cholesterol reduction on coronary atheromatous lesions is well documented.[9] Cholesterol-reducing drugs alone have a significant effect in preventing future bypass surgery, not to mention the added benefits of diet and smoking modification. Yet only a minority of patients who could benefit from these medications are prescribed them. Furthermore, the preventive effects of simple aspirin on myocardial infarction and of beta blockers on patients with a previous cardiac incident are also well documented but poorly subscribed to by physicians and patients. In the case of renal failure and diabetes, ACE inhibitors are preventive,[10] yet not adequately prescribed.

The current role of the medical director inside a managed care or utilization management organization was formulated around the policing strategy for this group of patients. A physician was needed who could understand if and how new procedures were relevant to diagnostic conditions, challenge the overuse of diagnostic and therapeutic interventions with the treating physicians, and relate this back to the benefit plan to determine if the beneficiary was covered under the terms of the plan. Medical directors' role in managed care plans has grown to include responsibility for quality, utilization management, physician credentialing, and plan accreditation preparation. Getting the job done with the most efficient use of resources is the new name of the game. Multiple procedures of questionable benefit have no value for anyone. Ensuring patients' adequate access, medication, compliance, information, and foresight serves all parties well. This has given rise to the new disease management industry, including companies who offer risk bearers (for the most part, managed care organizations) management support around these diseases. The leaders in this area are the PBMs and pharmaceutical manufacturers. They have direct access to physicians and patients through old marketing channels and PBM databases. Using medication properly for all of the right patients and ensuring compliance have enormous potential for increasing appropriate drug sales and for differentiating one's PBM services from competitors in an industry with very little real product differentiation. Device manufacturers too have needed to start thinking more about helping manage diseases as opposed to billing for units as their only avenue of survival.

However, the only management lever is at the patient-physician level. The value is all realized on the consequences of that interaction, and physicians have begun not only to realize and relish it but, more important, to organize around it. Medical specialists have created disease-based carve-out companies all over the country. They are contracting with those who own more global risk—managed care companies and wholly capitated provider groups. From cardiovascular disease to asthma, infectious disease to oncology, psychology to rehabilitation medicine, physicians are creating risk-bearing entities to receive capitation for their areas of disease expertise.

In this new world, the role of medical directors in managed care organizations changes. When disease risk is passed on to practitioners, helping physicians manage the risk through the provision of health care information and administrative support around the membership supplants policing activities. Since most full-time medical directors have been long separated from hands-on patient activities, pretensions of expertise around the actual care of patients lack credibility. Therefore, the role is reengineered to one of providing executive and technical informational support to the caregivers. These requisite skills are not those for which many of today's cadre of medical directors were recruited, and many of them will need additional training.

Group III: The 1%

These patients represent the true catastrophes in the health care delivery system. Afflicted with a significant primary diagnosis and usually one or more comorbidities, conflicting treatment plans from multiple providers, and resultant psychosocial and financial chaos, this group consumes a large amount of resources, yet has few management solutions. Such patients are the traditional outliers in the system, which payers accept are going to happen and around whom reinsurance is sometimes purchased. No two patients in this group with the exact same condition (severity adjusted) ever want to be treated the same way. Benefit plans are not written for these patients. Trying to fit them into these plans only creates problems.

The traditional management system for these patients (utilization review and case management) is a care-monitoring activity. The goal is to keep these extremely costly patients within the benefit plan whenever possible, avoid or deny leading-edge therapies not yet approved by external agencies as experimental, and ensure the lowest costs possible. At times, extraordinary benefits are allowed in lieu of costlier alternatives, as when extra home care visits are substituted for hospital inpatient services.

The case management philosophy applied to these patients grew out of the utilization management techniques developed for the less sick group II patients. There, illness is one-dimensional and focused on unique and discrete disease states, to which are applied sets of diagnostic and therapeutic procedures. For the very sick group III patients, disease protocols are necessary inputs, yet are insufficient to drive care management changes. These patients' problems are far more complex than simply diseases, and the solutions belie optimal disease protocols. The way the patients relate to the health care system is tied very closely to other factors such as family, culture, religion, and community. Unfortunately, when very ill with a plethora of technological options available at virtually no cost, these patients find themselves well into treatment plans that are unsatisfactory. For example, in the case of terminally ill patients, many die in places that were unintended.[6]

These complex and very ill patients are an important challenge for managed care organizations. Not only are they costly, but they are growing in number as the risk in new health care plans matures and as they begin to attract Medicare members who have a high incidence of complexity. Indeed, the incidence of complex patients in a Medicare population is anywhere from 7 to 10 times that in a commercial one (Franklin Health–Oxford Health Plan, Patient-Centered Care Pilot, unpublished data, 1996). The usual management strategy in closed networks of suppliers is to limit choices and reduce benefits. But forcing these square pegs into round holes has led to a significant public backlash against managed care companies as these patients and their families have resorted to lawyers and other means of public attention to help resolve their problems.

This situation is also not helpful to the patient-physician relationship. Here, physicians find themselves in the middle of a practical and moral dilemma. The services these patients require are often outside the attending physician's capabilities to provide them. Identifying the right team of physicians and ancillary providers, some of whom may not be a part of the managed care network of participating providers, can be a logistic feat for those who are engaged in a busy practice. Furthermore, with the rarity of some of the conditions, care should properly be obtained outside the plan. However, the authority to seek this care is relegated to another set of professionals inside the managed care organization. This further stresses what should be the pure advocacy role of the physician for the patient and strikes at the very heart of trust, or the patient's belief that the physician will not act in self-interest.

Ironically, cost reduction, quality improvement, and patient satisfaction can be achieved by a patient-led, patient-centered management strategy that fully informs patients about options for care and their consequences (Franklin Health–Oxford Health Plan, Patient-Centered Care Pilot, unpublished data, 1996; Franklin Health, internal data, 1996). Patients are not stupid. They make the right decisions even when confronted with complicated choices. Supporting them throughout to ensure proper execution of their decisions results in higher satisfaction with the benefit plan, subjectively improved quality of life, and reduced cost for the payer (Franklin Health–Oxford Health Plan, Patient-Centered Care Pilot, unpublished data, 1996; Franklin Health, internal data, 1996). Physicians are relieved, as once again they can feel that they are acting solely in the patient's interest.

Who will help physicians and risk bearers manage these patients is an unresolved industry issue. Managed care organizations firmly believe that these skills should be part of their core competency. However, they are burdened by the service site medical management infrastructure that grew around the old paradigm, and change will require a major organizational behavioral impetus. Additional skills are also necessary, particularly those related to epidemiology and measurement.

Possible new contributors are the health care reinsurers. As premium risk has been inexorably moving toward providers, what is today a small market providing insurance to capitated physicians on a per-member per-month fee basis for claims exceeding specific predefined thresholds is slated to grow to a $7 billion industry. Today, the only difference in what these reinsurers offer provider groups is difference in price. In the future, it is entirely possible that in addition to insurance, they will provide physicians with patient-centered management systems that will include software, patient identification and selection technology, data and epidemiological measurement support, and reporting capabilities. The net effect would be an entire system of risk management around the most complex patients in the risk pool. These patients would then be properly insured against catastrophe, and physicians would be removed from the inextricable ethical dilemma of being the insurer and the service provider at the same time.

CONCLUSION

Disease management is a simple term now used by many in the health care industry to describe a set of activities focused on patients and their illnesses. Its quick acceptance is representative of the insufficiencies resulting from the service-centered view, which was driven by a complicated set of economic, social, and professional issues.

With the new economics of health care, in which both healers and patients are reinvested in their relationship, the patient will once again assume his or her place as the main focus of the health care system. Physicians and hospitals will revert to their traditional responsibilities of providing value in the totality of illness.

The health care delivery system will necessarily reorganize to accommodate patient-centered values. In each segment of the industry, old players will reinvent themselves and new ones will emerge. Physicians will learn to manage properly their fiduciary responsibilities to patients. In doing so, they will successfully place limits on inappropriate risk assumption. They will also become far more efficient in the delivery of care than previously imaginable and will be able to articulate clearly the value they bring patients and populations. They will earn and deserve the trust of their patients.

Technological innovations will not be foisted on patients by pharmaceutical and device manufacturers through physicians. They will be driven by consumer knowledge and demand, and the health care industry will respond. Freedom of choice will emerge as a relentless force, particularly with the growing availability of medical information. As a direct result of this phenomenon, the public will not tolerate the delivery system being anything but patient-centered.

The return to traditional values in the health care delivery system is an enormous event in the evolution of the U.S. health care system. We have not yet come full circle and are still in the midst of a massive restructuring of the industry. Much of this is painful, but most of it will ultimately be beneficial.

References

1. Gray BH. Trust and trustworthy care in the managed care. *Health Aff.* 1997;16 (1):34–39.

2. Newcomer LN. Measures of trust in health care. *Health Aff.* 1997;16(1):50–51.

3. Beisecker AE, et al. Attitudes of medical students and primary care physicians regarding input of older and younger patients in medical decisions. *Med Care.* 1996;34:126–137.

4. Kaplan SH, et al. Characteristics of physicians with participatory decision-making styles. *Ann Intern Med.* 1996;124:497–504.

5. Kaplan SH, et al. Patient and visit characteristics related to physicians' participatory decision-making style. *Med Care.* 1995;33:1176–1187.

6. SUPPORT Principal Investigators. Care for seriously ill hospitalized patients. *JAMA.* 1995;274:1591–1598.

7. Fowles JB, et al. Taking health status into account when setting capitation rates. *JAMA.* 1996;276:1316–1321.

8. Wennberg JE, et al. Professional uncertainty and the problem of supplier-induced demand. *Soc Sci Med.* 1982;16:811–824.

9. Bjelajac A, et al. Prevention and regression of atherosclerosis: effect of HMG-CoA reductase inhibitors. *Ann Pharmacother.* 1996;30:1304–1315.

10. Brancati FL, et al. Epidemiology and prevention of diabetic nephropathy. *Curr Opin Nephrol Hypertens.* 1995;4:223–229.

Epilogue

Senator Bill Frist, MD

As we approach the millennium, we find ourselves in the midst of a health care revolution unlike anything we could have imagined. The old systems of medical and health care are eroding, and innovative ones are rapidly emerging. As these systems evolve, new and integrated approaches to care are being developed. Many factors have contributed to these changes, including increasing demands by the stakeholders for both cost containment and proof of quality and value. At the same time, advances in computer technology have provided us with the potential to develop centralized databases that can facilitate better provider and consumer decisions. Because of these changes, we are about to change the way we approach health promotion, disease prevention, and treatment.

Health care practitioners must reorient themselves if they are to meet the future challenges of our health care system. Specifically, practitioners must learn to use population-based data, as well as personal experience, for more informed health care decisions. Such a change is the basis of good practice. Today's stakeholders demand it. It is no longer just the physician and the patient, but also businesses, health plans, and the government who are at the table insisting that the management of the patient and his or her disease be both cost-effective and of high quality.

Disease management is not a new concept. Physicians have always managed disease, but they frequently did it as unconnected episodic events, never integrating all the elements of care that affect the results for a specific, at-risk patient population. These include prevention, education, monitoring of outpatient care, and follow-up after a hospital or office visit, to name but a few.

Source: Reprinted from a speech entitled, "Health Care Quality In a Time of Transition," by Senator Bill Frist, and the Prologue from *Disease Management: A Systems Approach to Improving Patient Outcomes,* by Warren Todd and David Nash, 1997, American Hospital Publishers, © Bill Frist.

Disease management might seem a simple concept, but it is a sophisticated approach to patient care that requires a knowledge of public health, disease history, health economics, and outcomes research. It integrates all these elements to produce for the population served the most cost-effective, continually improving, high-quality care available.

Modern disease management is information driven. Its cornerstone is quality outcomes research. If the right questions are not asked or the data are misinterpreted, much of the effort to improve a specific outcome will be misdirected. Care will be compromised, money poorly spent, and much labor wasted.

Yet this process goes far beyond mere outcomes research. The strength of effective disease management lies in the ability of an organization to integrate data from diverse reimbursement structures to measure the impact of resource coordination. The system must incorporate sound epidemiological methods to ensure quality health care. It should enable users to conduct resource planning, network development, evaluation, and management. Thus, the process is both information driven and continuously improved as more knowledge and health outcomes are analyzed and as more sophisticated evaluation tools are developed.

Such information about disease management and its quality will support the empowerment of consumers as well by enabling them to make truly informed decisions about their care. The impact of health informatics has already been felt in this area. The Internet has given many consumers the opportunity to form groups that provide support and share information about health care. Consumers are learning to assume more responsibility for their health care and the care of their loved ones. As they learn more about health care and ways to measure its quality, these stakeholders will become very important players at the table of disease management.

To sustain quality over the long term, we cannot ignore the basic building blocks that support it, namely, medical education and research. Likewise, we must not forget the institutions that bear the major responsibility for performance of these critical functions. Academic centers are unique and vulnerable establishments that must be safeguarded to allow for the adequate preparation of our next generation of practitioners and to provide a foundation for quality health care in the long term.

These and other quality-related questions (such as management of patient confidentiality and fraud) are important in the national health care debate. Legislative oversight must be provided if we are to develop a unified approach. Finally, where federal dollars are involved, as with Medicare and Medicaid, Congress has another, clear oversight role. In that role, it should stipulate that quality measurement and monitoring be an integral aspect of the health care system.

There are additional challenges. Cost is an issue. Computerization, video transfer of information, and broad familiarization with statistics will make analyses of outcome data increasingly easy, useful, acceptable, and powerful. Initially implementation of new data collection technologies can be expensive. However, a properly reformed system that includes a sophisticated information system to monitor enrollee utilization, patient access, physician practice patterns, and medical outcomes will greatly accelerate our ability to gather, analyze, and disseminate information. A system can then guide the individual physician as to the best way to manage a complex case. That is where cost savings will occur.

As useful information becomes available and efficiency improves, the cost of managing various diseases should drop. Some say that increased consumer access to information will reduce demand for services. However, it is difficult to predict the long-term trends in cost containment. As we learn to control the costs of the most visibly expensive diseases—as we eliminate the "fat in the system"—reductions in cost may level off.

The sheer number of players also makes efficient change difficult. The resolution of conflicts between incentives to expand access and those to lower costs must occur. Common standards must be universally accepted if we are to overcome barriers to the generation, translation, transfer, and storage of information. Evaluation tools must be shared.

Clearly, the federal government has several roles to play in the evolution of this young science:

1. The federal government must have an unwavering commitment to research and education programs that will continually improve the quality of care.

2. Government must support the continuing development of tools and techniques of quality measurement and improvement. It must insist that these tools and techniques be applied.

3. Government should assist in the coordination and collection of data so that there is greater uniformity in reporting. This is necessary so that consumers have the necessary tools to compare health plans based on quality, not just price.

4. Government must promote communication and education among all elements of society—public and private—about quality of care and quality measures. A common language about these issues must develop if we are to enable the public to communicate its concerns to policy makers and members of the industries that design information systems.

5. Government must guard patient confidentiality. By definition, improving the health and well-being of society's members will require the collection

of more comprehensive health data on individuals and populations (computer-based records). Quality initiatives and outcome measurement bring patient records, formerly the private domain of the physician-patient relationship, under outside third-party review. Today, there are inadequate federal protection laws, with different standards in different states.

6. We have a responsibility to protect against fraud and abuse that diverts scarce resources from the delivery of quality care. Although managed care no longer provides incentives to overutilize services, fraud will continue to pose a significant challenge to quality and the economic success of the health care market.

Disease management is never a finished product; it requires continuous reevaluation and introduction of changes in care. Therefore, these changes must be implemented incrementally. Everyone, including those from public and private sectors, consumers, providers, and payers, must have a place at the table. Vulnerable populations and institutions must also be involved. As medicine and our knowledge of facts that affect the health of our patients change, so will this process.

In the future, we will see a dramatic shift toward disease management and prevention, which holds great potential not only for alleviating human suffering but also for reducing costs. We will also see the further evolution of consumer empowerment. The same interests that brought us over-the-counter medicines, home test kits, prevention, and wellness are already making it possible for consumers to monitor their own health and communicate with providers through e-mail, video conferencing, and on-line self-help groups. Soon information that was once available only to medical professionals will be in reach of anyone with a computer and on-line service. In the future, to improve access and client satisfaction, we will also move health care facilities out into the communities where consumers live and work. Consequently we will produce greater numbers of satellite hospitals, community-based health centers, and other facilities that are located within areas of business, shopping, and "everyday" life.

How will these forces affect the larger view? As meaningful indicators become available, physicians will receive the feedback necessary to handle entire populations. They will learn to improve the health status of these groups in various ways visible to purchasers. Purchasers, in turn, will guide health care spending more efficiently once they have this information. Individual decision makers will also be empowered by the availability of information. With a growing consumer movement to guide them, consumers as well as purchasers will make more logical choices of health plans. Consequently, health care value will improve.

Thus we see that the next millennium will look very different from our current situation. As the system becomes more responsive to this evolving role, research priorities will be addressed more systematically. As providers learn to care for groups of patients, higher-risk populations will receive better care. Finally, as administrative overhead decreases, costs will drop. Providers, patients, and purchasers will be able to attack behavioral and environmental health issues. Community health in general will be addressed by a much more systematic and coordinated approach.

Our vision, then, is of a patient-centered health care system that employs leading-edge technologies in such a way as to enable providers and patients to shape a high-quality, cost-effective market. The government will play an oversight role in this process but must not be directly involved in the day-to-day management of patient care. Rather, its role is to ensure that systems that foster high-quality care are established in a systematic, unified way. Ultimately, market forces will empower consumers so that they and their physicians are once again making decisions about care.

Index

About the Editor

James B. Couch, M.D., J.D., FACPE is the Director-in-Charge of Coopers & Lybrand's worldwide Disease Management practice. Prior to that, he served as vice-president in charge of quality management at Travelers and as the medical director in charge of health care quality management nationally for MetLife. He has also served as an assistant professor (adjunct) at the University of Pennsylvania and Hahnemann University in Philadelphia. He has taught health policy, quality management and clinical decision analysis at those two universities, as well as Johns Hopkins, Cornell, N.Y.U., University of Connecticut, Yale, and Oxford (Green College). He served for three years (1992-1994) as the only physician Senior Examiner evaluating companies for the Malcolm Baldridge National Quality Award. His first book, "Health Care Quality Management for the 21st Century" was published in 1991 by the American College of Physician Executives and American College of Medical Quality.